# The Body at 40

# THE
# Body at 40

## Marjorie Shafto, M.D.
## and
## Gerald L. Hunt

*Illustration research by Pamela J. Mitsakos*

A PERIGEE BOOK

*For*
*Jennifer, Jonathan, and Fiona*

*For*
*Margaret Kathleen Carlin, a mother and a woman*
*of great substance, beauty, wit, and charm*

Perigee Books
are published by
The Putnam Publishing Group
200 Madison Avenue
New York, NY 10016

*Designed by Rhea Braunstein*

Library of Congress Cataloging-in-Publication Data

Shafto, Marjorie.
The body at forty.

"A Perigee book."
Includes index.
1. Middle aged women—Health and hygiene.   I. Hunt,
Gerald L.   II. Title. [DNLM: 1. Aging—popular works.
2. Health Promotion—popular works.   3. Women—
popular works. WA 590 S525b]
RA778.S545   1987     613'.04244      87-20238
ISBN 0-399-51378-7

Printed in the United States of America
2   3   4   5   6   7   8   9   10

# Acknowledgments

I was very fortunate to have parents who were enthusiastic when I decided to study medicine and who thought that I could accomplish whatever I set out to. My father, William Alexander Shafto, was a family doctor in the best tradition, an excellent diagnostician and a quiet humanitarian. My mother, Margaret Macdonald Shafto, an artist, was proud to see both her children become physicians.

I would like to acknowledge the School of Medicine of the University of Edinburgh, where some of my teachers were the finest in the world. And Professor Charles Roy Macdonald, my uncle, who delivered the first baby I ever saw brought into the world and who, with his wife Marjorie, was so wonderful to me when I was a medical student.

My patients over many years have taught me a great deal and I appreciate their loyalty and interest in my family. My friends have been steadfast and true: they are very special to me and they know who they are. And I'm grateful to my family, who never minded when I rushed out to deliver a baby at Thanksgiving or Christmas; my daughters learned to get the turkey on the table. I am very lucky to have three interesting and terrific children who are enormous fun to be with. Last, I would like to thank my brother, Alan, with whom I have shared a practice for so many years, for his quiet, loyal support. He is a caring and compassionate physician, who is totally devoted to his family and his patients. He and his wife Patty, their children Keith and Jackie, and my own three children are my constant source of joy.

The inspiration for this book must be credited to our editor, Judy Linden, who has that special strength of heart and will that makes a truly great editor. And with friends like Adele Leone and Richard Monaco of the Adele Leone Agency, Inc., . . . who needs agents?

Lee Harrison contributed expert researching skills and writing to the text of the original manuscript and we are in his debt. And Susan Philipson, copy editor, did a terrific job.

Appreciation is expressed to Dennis Neeld for his editorial guidance, and to Martina Vera for her patience.

A very special thank you to Colette Michelle Crean, who, in effect, this book is all about.

# Contents

# Introduction

If you are approaching forty this year you are a product of the baby boom. You were born just after the end of World War II, probably in 1946 or 1947. You were a child of the fifties and a teenager of the sixties. The Beatles, flower children dancing in the California sunshine, the sexual revolution—these were all part of your youth. And the tragic reality of the Kennedy assassination is, like acid on metal, permanently etched on your memory.

Life in America in the eighties is exciting: women are benefiting from opportunities available to them in education, personal development and professional careers, and they have the freedom to choose among many different life-styles. The women's movement has enabled thousands of women to be liberated from the rigid roles prescribed for them by society for generations and has opened doors into many previously exclusively male domains. By the age of forty, many of you have taken advantage of these new options and have settled down to live them.

Many of you chose to marry early and now your childbearing years are behind you. Your families are well launched; your offspring are fast approaching adult life and independence, leaving you free for the first time in years to spend some time on yourself, to go back to school, start a new job, take up a career, or fulfill some secret ambition. Your newfound freedom tastes sweet. Some of you may be struggling in unhappy marriages or coping with the pain of divorce and the difficulties of single parenthood. Some of you have chosen a "singles" life-style that is comfortable and right for you. Career women who put off marriage and spent long years educating and establishing themselves in responsible positions are now possibly juggling full-time jobs, marriage, and young children, along with their myriad physical and emotional needs. "Having it all" calls for enormous energy.

Whatever your status, have you stopped to assess *your* needs? The years ahead should be the best of your life—the most productive and, in many ways, the most fun! Your health should be at its peak. The media do women a great disservice by intimating that life after forty is all downhill. The emphasis our culture places on youth as a synonym for beauty is reinforced by fashion illustrations using adolescents for models and advertisements describing treatment for problems of "over twenty-three skin." But take a look at the Catherine Deneuves and Elizabeth Taylors of this world! As more of us than ever before enter our mature years, hopefully the pendulum will swing toward admiration for the loveliness of a poised, confident woman in her forties or fifties. The increasing appearance of older women in movie and TV roles is certainly a good sign!

Turning forty should be a triumph, a cause of celebration. Like Miss Jean Brodie, you are entering your prime. To maintain that prime, you must think seriously about your present health and future well-being. It is a time to pause, reflect, take stock, and, if necessary, plan to make changes in your lifestyle that will keep you in the best of health for the wonderful years ahead. You need to know what to expect in the future and what to do to make sure that your body will continue to meet the demands you'll be placing on it. You need knowledge—up-to-date medical information about your body, its functioning, its needs, its idiosyncracies. There are many sources of information—in fact, so many books and articles that it can become very confusing. Which diet, you ask, shall I try first? What about the Pill at my age? What are the chances of my getting breast cancer? How can I prevent those change-of-life problems with which I saw my mother struggle?

This book will give you sound information about all these topics and more, geared specifically to your age: facts about your skin, hair, and figure; facts about the wonders (yes, forget all those horror stories) of menopause, about hormone treatment, about birth control and sexual activity and the new freedoms that come with forty. You'll also learn about those public enemies number one and two—cancer and heart attack—and about that "delicate" subject, venereal disease. Might it be too late, you wonder, to change self-destructive behavior to a life-style that will improve the quality and length of your life? The answer is a definite no!

*The Body at 40,* while explaining the functioning of your body, will suggest ways of slowing aging processes as much as possible. With women's increasing longevity (the average is now seventy-seven years for a female baby born today), most of us will live a total number of years after menopause that only a century ago would have been considered entire lifetimes. You will need to know about osteoporosis—the loss of bone mass from your body—and its risk factors, and in particular, ways to keep your bones in positive calcium balance. This means that you need information about nutrition. The old saying "You are what you eat" is true, and in these pages you will find information on your "ideal" weight and ways in which to achieve this goal by diet and exercise.

Exercise—do you know what kind is best for you? Best for your heart? your lungs? Which is better for preventing osteoporosis—bicycling, swimming, or running? It's important that any energy you expend be channeled in the right direction.

Birth control is something about which you have already made decisions. But methods suitable for you in your twenties and thirties may not be appropriate in your forties. The latest heartening news about the Pill, (not in its role as a contraceptive) is eye-opening. How about sterilization? It's the final solution for many women of our age who decide they definitely do not want any more children. A "change-of-life" baby, even if unplanned, can be a blessing; however, you should know your options.

If you marry at forty, of course you still have time to have a family, but don't put it off too long—and do discuss it with your doctor before attempting to become pregnant.

Estrogen therapy during menopause—the pros and the cons—is an important and fascinating topic to mull over with your doctor. Forearmed with knowledge of the latest developments, you'll know the right questions to ask your physician when it comes to deciding how to handle your gynecological health.

Cancer is a subject of enormous concern to women our age, and today there is a wealth of information available as research progresses on the various forms of the disease. Do you know what risk factors are associated with breast cancer and when to start having mammograms, or soft-tissue X rays of the breasts? Could you be a candidate for cervical cancer? Do you know what recently developed tests are available for its detection? How about the telltale early warning signs of ovarian cancer—the recently discovered signals every woman in her forties should watch for? Colon cancer: did you realize you're now at a crucial age? You'll learn the answers to these questions and more in our special section on cancer and the body at forty.

A most important part of your plan to stay healthy for the years ahead is to discover as much as you can about your family history. Your doctor may have asked about your family's health—probably when you were pregnant—and now's the time to update that information. Knowing the causes of death of your grandparents, and even great-grandparents, and other relatives can be of immense value to you; armed with such information, your doctor can advise you on blood tests that can spot any tendencies toward these illnesses or conditions while there is still time to do something about them. Don't forget that medical knowledge has increased enormously and that many conditions are treatable, especially if diagnosed early. So talk to family members about health!

Do you know the full effects of alcohol, drugs, and smoking on your body? Are you aware of the effect on your lungs of other people's smoking? Do you know how much alcohol is a liver poison? Most important, do you know that it is not too late to change your addictive behavior to minimize damage?

Over the years, I have seen many changes in medicine and in the way women view themselves. Some of the changes I laud have been ones that revert to more traditional ways, especially with regard to childbirth and the rearing of infants. The changes I have seen among my female patients I also applaud: a distinct eagerness to understand their own bodies as they grow through life; less of a tendency to take things for granted, to leave everything up to their physician and simply wait for checkup time. The new woman in her forties *wants* to be informed and she *will* question the advice she receives on her own body. This is extremely sensible and very healthy, and I'm all for it. That's why this book came about—because the majority of women who come into my office want to know more about their physical selves.

The first thing you should know is how resilient, adaptable, and strong the female body is. In fact, you'd probably be surprised to learn just how tough we really are. I speak from personal experience: I was a third-year medical student—and one of the youngest medical students in the country—when I and several others embarked on a salt-crusted old ferry to cross the Irish Sea from Scotland to Ireland on a cold St. Patrick's Day. We were going to deliver babies to women in their homes in the poorer sections of Dublin. We were to be their only resource when they went into labor. I was armed with enormous enthusiasm and a black leather doctor's bag packed with sponges, sutures, antiseptic solution, rubber gloves, and obstetrical forceps. A textbook of midwifery (the British still use this term in preference to "obstetrics") was in my suitcase. I had seen a few women give birth and had scrubbed in the delivery room and studied the labor diagrams very carefully. But this was to be the real thing!

In Ireland I learned something very important from mothers who had experienced childbirth a dozen times and more: for the woman left mostly to her own (and the midwife's) devices, having babies is no big deal. No clinical and sterile surroundings, no special anesthetics or painkillers; they just did what came naturally—and took it uncomplainingly in their stride.

It has been my privilege to deliver babies to all kinds of mothers since those early days—mothers of different religions and ethnic backgrounds and ranging in age from fourteen to forty-seven. When I started practice in Connecticut, I was amazed to find that most women were delivered with spinal anesthesia and forceps and that breast-feeding was not in fashion. I was always very keen to emphasize to a first-time mother that childbirth is a natural procedure and that nursing a baby is easy and a most rewarding experience. My copy of Dr. Grantley Dick Read's book *Childbirth Without Fear* was borrowed and enjoyed by dozens of patients, going back to the late fifties. It proved to me the value of a book and women's eagerness to know more about physical processes.

I have seen a generation of women grow up, go to work or to college, become career women, writers, professionals, marry and start their own families. Now I deliver babies to some of these young women I brought into the world. It has been exciting to look after these women, to support them through difficult times, to listen to their problems and help them with their families.

14

My own three children were born over the years and I had personal experience of pregnancies, Cesarean births, "terrible twos," and all the wonderful stages of childhood and adolescence. So much happiness—and, of course, some pain also. Through these busy years of medical practice and my own family life, I continued to find that most women are very competent in handling pregnancies, illness, and problems with both older parents and children.

I repeat: women *do* have tremendous resiliency, which enables most of us to survive the death of loved ones, divorce, and disabling illness with courage and strength, to hold down jobs, bring up children, and somehow manage to remain optimistic about what the future may bring. Women can be helped to cope when they know as much of their own biology, their makeup, as possible. Understanding the changes in their bodies at puberty, in pregnancy, at menopause, and in the later years allows women to adapt better, to change their habits to more beneficial ones, and to live their lives in maximum comfort and with maximum energy for the tasks facing them.

This book is written specifically for women who have gone beyond the early years of growth, self-discovery, and finding their place in society. By following the advice on these pages, not only will you have more healthful years ahead in which to enjoy your work, leisure, and family; you will also be setting an excellent example for your children.

Your doctor's years of experience, knowledge, and concern are fountains of wisdom from which you can draw as you enter these exciting years. In *The Body at 40,* you'll discover ways of supplementing your doctor's care; there is much you can do to help yourself. An intimate knowledge of your body and its workings can put you on the right path to optimal health for the rest of your life.

And remember, hitting forty is just the beginning!

# 1
# Where Am I Now?

Now that you are in your forties, it would be wise to stop and assess where you are in time and how you are in terms of your body's structure and function. My training as a doctor tends to make me very systematic, so let's discuss your body's structure, or anatomy, first, then its functioning, or physiology. Keep in mind that a good deal of your present appearance and fitness depends on both your heredity and what sort of stresses your body has been subjected to.

Heredity is one thing we can't plan. However, because we are so genetically intertwined with our forebears, knowledge about them—specifically about their physical health—can help us build a pretty accurate blueprint of what to expect for ourselves (see the section on family history in Chapter 6).

The body of a dancer or an athlete who has been concerned with good diet and exercise for the past twenty years or so will naturally be different from that of a woman with a less physically demanding life-style. They can all, however, enjoy excellent health. Then there's the extreme case of the woman of sedentary habits, who has a longstanding problem with overweight, indulges in a poor diet, and has not sought adequate medical care; she's obviously going to be in relatively poor shape as far as overall health is concerned. However, it's *never* too late to change. In fact, forty is an ideal age to abandon bad habits and start tuning and toning the wonderful female machine—even if it means some rather drastic changes. Remember what I said earlier about the female body's resilience and adaptability to change? Maybe now's the time for you to test this out.

Where are you in time? You're in the prime of your life! Of that you can be sure. While it may be natural to feel a little sadness that youth is behind you, to feel some nostalgia for the enthusiasms of your twenties, it is important to believe that the years ahead hold the promise of further exciting adventures and satisfactions.

Think about this: many of you have more than forty years still to live to the fullest. Why not make the most of them, make every one count, and be in the best physical health to enjoy the riches that await you. What you have now is very precious—maturity. You have learned an enormous amount about yourself—your capabilities, talents, strengths, and endurance. You have learned your weaknesses (we all have them) and how to adjust to or camouflage them. You have learned how to make the best of your appearance by choosing colors and styles carefully. You know much more about relationships with other people, both men and women, than you did in the past. Hopefully, you enjoy self-confidence and feel free to express your opinions about matters that are important to you. The views of a mature woman are a force to be reckoned with. Just remember how much you used to look up to your mother's maturity and knowledge when you were young. Today *you* make the sensible choices for your dependents after wisely considering the options that only a mature mind can recognize. You feel good about yourself. This is not just a pep talk. Stop and think about all this.

As good a place as any to start our tour of the body in prime time is the head.

## THE BRAIN

The ultimate control center; the most sophisticated flight deck in the world. A computer will probably never be invented that has the flexibility, dexterity, and awesome power of the human brain. It is the one organ of our body that, discounting disease or injury, will continue to improve with the years, just like a fine wine. True, each day we lose a few more brain cells to the aging process, but many neurologists specializing in the function of the brain will swear that we use only a fraction of the organ's billions of cells anyway.

Your brain will continue to improve its performance as long as you continue to prime it with information. It's the one organ in the body that can never be overloaded with work. It is reassuring for us all that more research than ever is being devoted to the mysteries of the human brain, to its complex chemistry and role in the central nervous system. Changes in the brain occur during our entire life span. Believe it or not, the brain actually begins to start aging when you are in your twenties, but no more than a 5 percent decrease in total brain weight can be expected until you are well into your seventies and eighties.

For many women, the forties may bring stressful life situations: a booming career, children who are going through the stormy teenage years or are ready to fly the coop (the empty-nest syndrome), or, of course, with the ever-increasing divorce rate, a time of instability while we marshal our resources. But don't let anyone tell you that this type of stress can deteriorate your brain. There has never been any proven scientific connection between stress and loss of mental capacity and greatly diminished brain cells. If anything, stress handled constructively and with confidence can only help to improve the brain's vast store of knowledge.

The only danger your brain may face at this time in life is the remote possibility of a stroke, and for that to happen, vascular disease must be present. Cerebrovascular (brain blood vessel) disease accounts for some 160,000 deaths a year and is the third leading cause of death nationally for both sexes. However, a woman in her forties is not in the critical age range for risk of a stroke. A stroke is the result of a stoppage or a slowdown of blood to the brain. It can be the direct result of high blood pressure and changes of atherosclerosis, or plaque formation, in the arteries supplying the head and neck.

You must be concerned with your cholesterol, lipid or fatty acid levels, and blood pressure. You must exercise and eat well, not just to prevent heart disease but to promote clear thinking through good blood flow to the brain. Let's keep those little gray cells functioning at a fast clip!

A word of encouragement. Although as we get older we cannot expect our memory to improve or our neurological functioning to increase in efficiency, remember that our constantly enlarging experience of life and wonderful warehouse of memories help us to become more creative and better at problem solving and organizing than ever before—and more valuable to others in the process.

## THE EYES

Your eyes are the most expressive part of your body; they allow you to reach out to the rest of the world and life to reach in to your brain. However, these wonderful orbs are not immune to change.

In my thirties, and being nearsighted, I thought Ha! one of the advantages of entering my forties will be throwing away my faithful glasses. Well, guess who's wearing bifocals now! With age, we tend to have more difficulty accommodating or

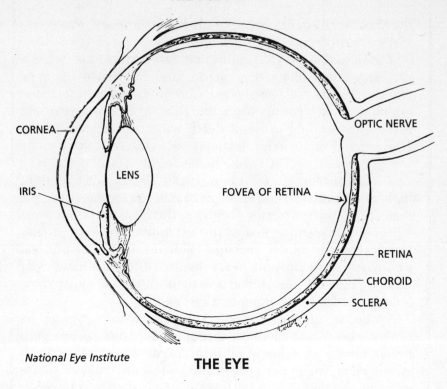

CORNEA

IRIS

LENS

OPTIC NERVE

FOVEA OF RETINA

RETINA

CHOROID

SCLERA

*National Eye Institute*     **THE EYE**

focusing on close objects. This is due to a gradual change in the elasticity of the lens that affects the eye's focus. (Naturally, if you're farsighted to begin with, you'll become more so with age.)

The lens of the eye, whose shape determines (again through heredity) whether you have 20/20 vision, myopia (nearsightedness), or hyperopia (farsightedness), thickens and becomes less elastic as we age. Inevitably, it becomes increasingly difficult for your eye muscles to bend the lens to bring close-up objects into focus: this is called presbyopia. Just be glad, if you have to wear glasses, that our modern eyepieces are so stylish.

While we're discussing eyewear, if you have not tried contact lenses yet and need corrective glasses, why not try them now? They can give you a whole new look, especially now that tinted ones are available. Today you can get bifocal contact lenses and also "extended-wear" lenses, which do not have to be removed while you sleep. Although you may be told they can be worn for as long as two weeks at a stretch, I always recommend that they be changed and cleaned weekly to reduce any risk of irritation. The latest developments in contact lenses make them easy to insert, wear, and care for.

If you look closely at your eyes in a mirror, you may see a white circle just on the outside of the iris where it meets the sclera, or white part of the eyeball. This is called the arcus senilis and, despite the sound of it, is nothing to worry about. More noticeable in dark-eyed people, this opaque ring is just another sign of aging. However, no matter how good you feel your eyesight may be, your forties is a good time to have a professional eye exam, by an optometrist or ophthalmologist, that includes testing for glaucoma (see below).

When the eye doctor examines your eyes with an ophthalmoscope, he sees your optic nerve, the only part of your brain visible from outside the body. He can view the tiny blood vessels, or capillaries, of the retina. As these can be changed in appearance by certain conditions, hypertension and diabetes among others, this examination is of value for more than just your eyes. Any alterations in the size or shape of your pupil, or in its ability to contract when exposed to light, are clues every doctor looks for. They can be telltale signs for many conditions, from concussion after a head injury to a neurological problem. It's interesting to note that 15 percent of "normal" people have pupils of different sizes. Only if pupil size suddenly changes should you be concerned and seek a professional opinion. Obviously, it is prudent to investigate with your doctor any difficulties of vision or pain in the eyes. And, of course, there are certain problems we should pay particular attention to, such as those discussed below.

21

## DIABETES AND THE EYE

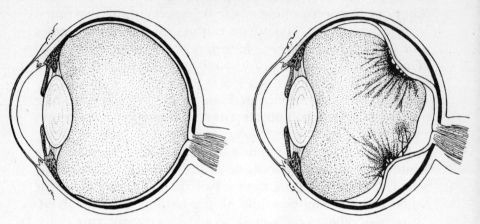

Cross-sectional view of a normal eye (left) and an eye with diabetic retinopathy (right). In this disorder, new blood vessels may grow into the vitreous—the normally clear fluid filling the eye's interior. These abnormal vessels bulge, leak fluid, and occasionally rupture. Bleeding within the retina can cause scarring and retinal distortion, eventually producing serious loss of vision or blindness. *The Upjohn Company*

# Glaucoma

A disease in which the fluid inside the eye exerts too much pressure, glaucoma is often inherited: there is an approximate 10 percent prevalence among first-degree relatives. Having increased ocular or internal eye pressure does not mean that you have high blood pressure, although hypertension may be a risk factor for glaucoma, which is the cause of 12 percent of the cases of blindness in the United States.[1] As there are often no warning signs of glaucoma, it may cause damage to your eyes before you are aware of it.

About 1 million people in the United States have glaucoma, and there have been many campaigns by service organizations for people to get exams *before* the condition gets serious. Don't wait until you are in your fifties; go for an eye test now. Glaucoma does not have to be a problem. Treatments, I'm happy to report, are getting more sophisticated and more successful every year. Sometimes eye drops will keep the pressure within normal boundaries; if not, oral medications and, most recently, laser treatments, in addition to traditional surgery, are all extremely successful.

The clue to effectively treating glaucoma is early diagnosis: danger signals are seeing halos around lights, especially when you are driving at night, and pain in the eye. Again, glaucoma can be diagnosed only by tonometry—measuring the pressure in the eye. Don't neglect this vital examination.

## Cataracts

The other common condition that interferes with vision is cataracts. These are unusual at our age, but you should know about them. For reasons not yet fully understood, areas of the lens become opaque, so that vision is altered as light enters the eye. In the beginning the condition can be helped by the use of special glasses, but eventually near-normal vision is restored by the surgical removal of the natural lens and the insertion of an artificial one. This has been truly one of the miracles of modern medicine.[2]

Cataract surgery used to be considered a risky and even dangerous procedure. Today it is safe—with a 95 percent success rate—and is usually performed on an outpatient basis. The use of modern lens implants allows most patients to instantly regain near-normal vision. With such favorable prospects, should cataract victims immediately rush into surgery? No! Patients need to make their own decision, based on a number of considerations. Except in very rare cases, a cataract may be left alone until visual impairment starts to cause problems. The eyes are not damaged by leaving the cataract in place for a while; nor is the potential improvement in vision from a lens implant reduced by waiting. In fact, as cataracts grow very slowly—and require no ongoing medical treat-

23

ment—it's often possible to wait ten to twenty years before visual impairment makes surgery necessary.

As a rule of thumb, I suggest delaying surgery until one or more of the following occurs:

- You can no longer pass a driver's test or drive safely.
- Reading, writing, or watching TV becomes difficult.
- Significant loss of depth perception occurs.
- Vision is reduced in bright sunlight or darkness.

Surgery usually takes less than an hour and is performed under a local anesthetic. During the following six to eight weeks, it may be advisable to wear a patch over the eye at night and to avoid physical straining, such as lifting heavy objects, which can put pressure on blood vessels in the eye. Intraocular lens implants (IOLs) are the most popular replacement lens today: unlike contact lenses, they're permanent, generally can't be felt, and require no care. If visual or rejection problems occur, doctors are now able to change the lens until one is found that's just right.

## Pinkeye

Its medical name is "conjunctivitis." This is an infection of the conjunctiva, or lining of the eye, which is common at any age and is treated by your doctor with specific drugs, depending on whether it is viral or bacterial in origin. The condition can be very infectious, so be careful not to share towels with others in the household.

Dryness of the conjunctiva can be a problem for those of us over forty whose work involves reading fine print, checking columns of small figures, or working long hours at video-display terminals. The eyes need to rest between hours of visual work. If eye drops don't solve the problem, you should consult an ophthalmologist, who may prescribe drugs if necessary. He should also discuss with you the possibility of its being an allergic condition and make recommendations accordingly. Dry eyes, unfortunately, can also be a symptom of rheumatoid arthritis and may require long-term treatment with eye drops.

One word about eye makeup. Women can become allergic to cosmetics, even the ones they've been using for years. So, if you have itching or scaling of the eyelids or around the eyes, consider your makeup as the most likely cause. Also remember that liquid cosmetics are quite a breeding ground for bacteria. If you have an infection on your face, you can reinfect yourself from your foundation or moisturizer or liquid eye cosmetics.

## THE EARS

Your hearing—what a wonderful system it is! The first thing you should know is good news: women are less prone to deafness than men and, as a matter of fact, only about 20 percent of women in their late sixties have hearing problems that are significant.

Although it is unlikely at your age to have any age-related hearing loss, you should be aware that some diminution of your powers of hearing has been going on since your mid-thirties. If you have been blasted with loud rock music or industrial noise for some time, then your hearing may well be impaired already.

A temporary hearing loss can be caused by blockage of the ear canal with wax or by a collection of fluid in the middle ear as a result of an infection. This is particularly common in women who suffer from allergies. These conditions should be treated promptly. There are many causes of deafness which are progressive, so at the slightest hint of trouble, contact an ear-nose-and-throat specialist to ensure that you are doing all you can to preserve your hearing.

# THE NOSE

Our sense of smell usually works beautifully any old time. It is the sense that is disturbed least by the aging process.

Temporary problems are usually related to the mucous membrane, or lining of the nose, which can dry out and get infected or develop growths called polyps. These conditions usually respond well to treatment. I have had a few patients over the years who decided they hated their noses and elected to undergo plastic (or, as most practitioners prefer to call it, "cosmetic") surgery in their forties. Why? Probably because by the age of forty many women simply decide it's a good time to try a new look. Reconstruction surgery has been refined to an art, and there are many fine surgeons today performing minor miracles on women's profiles. Cosmetic surgery can be expensive, but it is within reach of many more women than was the case years ago (see Chapter 3).

# THE MOUTH AND TEETH

We are indeed fortunate to live in a part of the world where dentistry is extremely sophisticated and highly successful in preserving our teeth, usually for a lifetime.

Many of you will have had good dental care for years, but I would emphasize that proper dental hygiene becomes more and more important as you get older. Effects of aging on the tooth structure itself are minimal—the enamel becomes thinner and stained yellow—but excessive bone loss or osteoporosis in later life can cause the teeth to loosen in the jaw. The biting surfaces of the teeth are ground down a little, but that is to be expected after so many years of continuous eating. If your diet has been good and your bite is normal, then your teeth should be in good shape. By the way, that old saying "getting long in the tooth" is a truism. Your teeth may well look a little longer than they did a few years back, but that is because the gum line tends to recede as we age.

The biggest single problem we encounter in our mouth is with the gums. Some recession is acceptable, but inflammation—what is called gingivitis—is the major cause of loss of teeth. Perfectly good teeth can be lost when the supporting structures become infected. I find that I can spot gingivitis before a woman begins to have problems with bleeding gums, puffiness and soreness, and obvious infections between the gums and teeth. Use a good mirror and inspect your teeth and gums carefully. The gums should be a healthy pink and not puffy. If you see swelling or a dull redness in the tissue, do not hesitate to see your dentist at once. Proper care can save your teeth.

I'm sure you've seen women of our age wearing braces and have wondered about it. New discoveries show that proper alignment of teeth by means of braces not only improves esthetic appearance but also promotes a much healthier mouth and provides for teeth that will be less prone to structural problems later in life.

Today there is far less dental decay than was seen years ago, due mainly to better diets, less chewing of gum and fewer sweets, and the introduction of fluoride—into our drinking water and toothpaste and topically applied during dental visits. Add to that improved techniques and materials used in filling teeth, and the latest use of wonderful new synthetics for crowns, bridges, and bonding, and you can see why there is no reason we shouldn't keep a million-dollar smile for life.

To those of you who have not been to a dentist recently, I would suggest two things: one, *go,* and two, don't worry about pain! Most of us are chickens when it comes to dental work, but don't let that prevent you from getting the excellent care now available. I have personally had pain-free drillings, fillings, and root-canal work, and can attest to the wonder-working properties of Novocain. Increasingly sophisticated tools, too—finely honed high-speed drills, for example—make the dental experience far less intimidating than in the past.

## THE VOICE

Have you noticed that your voice has become slightly deeper, maybe a little huskier during the past few years? Don't worry: this doesn't mean you are taking on masculine tendencies. It's yet another, but harmless, female twist of aging.

The muscles and ligaments that make up the voice box and surrounding tissues change character with age. They become less elastic, and this affects the pitch of the voice. Inevitably we women find our voices becoming deeper. In the years to come, the vocal cords can even bend or bow, and this leads to the wavering voice we often associate with the elderly.

There is one thing you must be aware of: these changes in the vocal pattern are very gradual. A sudden huskiness or hoarseness of the voice is a sign that you should seek immediate medical attention. Severe changes in vocal tone can indicate polyps on the vocal cords, hyperthyroidism, and even cancer. It's not worth taking the risk to ignore a problem that is often treatable if taken care of early. Don't neglect changes in your voice.

## THE BREASTS

Few of us are ever satisfied with the shape of our breasts. Our breast-oriented culture is mostly to blame for what, with some women, borders on the paranoid: we would like our breasts to be bigger or smaller, more rounded or less so. But, ladies, whether we like it or not, apart from obesity, the shape and size of our breasts is usually (once again) part of our genetic makeup.

The amount of glandular tissue in the breasts tends to diminish as we enter our forties, but this is often replaced by fat.

28

Women ask me if they can restore their breasts to a youthful trimness by exercising. Here are the facts: there are no muscles in the breasts, except around the nipples, so exercising can do nothing for the tone of your breasts. Exercise builds up the pectoral muscles on which the breasts lie but will not raise the breasts on the chest wall. I tell adolescents and young women always to wear a good supporting bra especially when exercising or pregnant; this is usually much more comfortable than going braless. Weight loss may reduce the fatty content of the breast and so alter the contour.

It's not realistic to expect the breasts to stay exactly the same over the years, especially if you are heavy or if you have been pregnant and nursed a baby. Some women seem to be smaller after they have finished nursing, but basically once the ligaments above the breast have been stretched, they will stay stretched. Wearing good-quality undergarments is helpful, and women who feel uncomfortable with their breasts at night might want to consider wearing a nightgown with a built-in bra.

Breast augmentation, or surgery to increase the breast size, is often very successful. Methods and materials for insertion into the breast and breast area to achieve the desired effect are constantly changing. My best advice is to choose a plastic surgeon carefully and discuss the procedure and cost thoroughly before you take the plunge. I can say that results are usually excellent, but you must understand that there will be scars. Breast augmentation is a marvelous new technique that makes women feel much more comfortable with their bodies.

Breast reduction is rather different. Many women with large breasts have a lot of pain premenstrually, constant backaches, and deep imprints in their shoulders from their bra straps. They are often unable to run or exercise without discomfort. More often than not, reduction of the breasts is done to relieve pain and to allow a woman to exercise for good health. This fact alone indicates that breast reduction for the purpose of relieving pain is much more apt to be paid for by your insurance than if it were purely for cosmetic reasons.

29

I have seen several women drop to a bra-cup size much more appropriate for their height and weight after surgery, buy nice new bras, and take off happily to aerobics classes or the tennis courts.

## THE STOMACH/ABDOMEN

Obviously, the state of your abdominal wall, its flatness and leanness, is dependent on what your history has been in terms of pregnancies, surgical operations, *and* obesity. But it is *also* quite certain that if your tummy is flabby and you no longer have taut, firm muscles, you can regain a lot of tone and trimness by exercising.

Our tummy is where we have an advantage over the male physique. Whereas most men, when they put on weight, tend to carry it around the belt line, we women will spread extra weight out more evenly around the trunk. The catch here is: we also get extra on the thighs and buttocks!

The best exercises for firming up the tummy are sit-ups, leg raises, and bicycling. But they need to be done regularly and for a specific duration. There are excellent exercise programs on TV, so you can make a good start exercising on a daily basis in the comfort of your own home, even if you cannot get to an aerobics class or gym.

Exercise definitely helps flatten your tummy, both by weight loss and by strengthening the abdominal muscles.

## THE BUTTOCKS

Have you been looking at that sagging derriere recently and has the thought crossed your mind that it might be time to buy a girdle? After all, Mother and Grandmother used to wear one, didn't they? Don't. Wearing girdles is not a good idea at any age. They can do more damage than good. A girdle may give you a trimmer look, but in effect it is supporting those slack underlying muscles and further increasing the tendency for them to become lazy and saggy. There's only one way to trim the behind and firm up the front, and that's with the appropriate exercise.

Any kind of leg exercise that stretches the muscles of the buttocks will help firm up your bottom. Don't let anyone tell you that a sagging posterior has to be part-and-parcel of being forty. There is absolutely no reason why you shouldn't have the buttocks of a twenty-year-old. It's only a matter of muscle tone and exercise.

## THE SPINE

Yes, we do get shorter with age. If you were able to look at X rays that were taken of your spine in your twenties and compare them with ones taken today, you'd see a noticeable difference. The simple reason we are losing height is that our spine has become more compacted with age; the vertebrae and discs in between them have shrunk somewhat. This is all part of the natural process of aging and there's not much you can do about it.

We also have a tendency to stoop forward with age. This is again due to a physiological change in the makeup of the spine. The front part of the vertebrae tends to compact more than the rear, and this throws the entire posture slightly forward. Although this may not have been noticeable during your thirties, the seeds were being sown and it will become slightly more apparent now that you are in your forties.

There *are* preventive measures you can take now. Make sure that you are getting an adequate daily supply of calcium. This is most important—in fact, *vital*—at your stage of life. If you want to avoid the ravages of osteoporosis (discussed in Chapter 6), the best time to start prophylactic measures is *now*.

While you may not be able to stop the spine from its natural progression of aging, you can improve your posture by building strong abdominal muscles. Again, it is of tremendous value

31

to have superstrong tummy muscles. If you care about your back and want to prevent the inevitable aches and often chronic severe pain associated with a degenerating spine, combine good nutrition and adequate calcium with exercise to strengthen the abdominal muscles. It may be hard work, but it's well worth it in the long run.

## THE LEGS AND FEET

If you have had a tendency to gain weight during your thirties, there's little doubt that some of it will have settled on your thighs and legs. Of all the "cosmetic" complaints I hear from my patients, most concern the thighs. Nobody wants to walk around with saddlebag thighs. Unless you've put on weight, there's no reason why your thighs and calves shouldn't be approximately the same shape they were in when you were in your twenties.

There's also such a thing as overreaction to the shape your legs are in. Chances are that if you haven't put on the odd extra pounds since your twenties or thirties, and you enjoy a reasonably active life-style, there's no reason to think that your legs are giving out on you. I don't know why, but many women just seem to expect their legs to go downhill after forty. Most often the sad shape your legs are in is all a state of mind. Think and look positively, and if you are still not satisfied, remember that there are all sorts of wonderful fancy new styles and textures of pantyhose out there that visually slim down and bring more appealing contours to the legs.

As for feet, yes, women do have more problems than men. It's hardly surprising, though, considering some of the footwear we torture our poor *pieds* with. Wearing heels that put us one to four inches above terra firma for twenty or thirty years not only wrecks our natural posture but also puts undue pressure on the bones of our feet.

High-heeled shoes tend to have wafer-thin soles, and this can result in excessive pressure on the metatarsal bones—and pain around the ball of the foot. Calluses—ugly raised hard patches of skin—can also develop. Women concerned about pretty feet may be tempted to remove calluses, but before you do, remember one thing: those calluses are nature's way of building protection at a trouble spot. If you are going to continue wearing the same shoes that sparked the calluses, no matter how many times you smooth them down with strokes of a pumice stone, they're just going to grow back again. It is best to treat calluses at the first sign of trouble. Buy a metatarsal support pad and place it between the shoe and the affected area.[3]

Bunions are another common female foot problem. Although these bony outgrowths probably began developing when you were a teenager, it is now in your forties when they may be presenting a real problem. Bunions should be removed surgically only if they are causing pain. You can keep more comfortable by wearing properly fitting shoes. A bunionectomy is surgical removal of the excess bony tissue and realignment of the great toe, which is usually very successful and well worth considering. Traditional surgery may put you off your feet for some weeks but there are amazing new techniques in foot and toe surgery that require a minimal incision through which a surgeon guides a "roto-rooter"-type instrument to the trouble spot to grind down the excessive bone growth. The unwanted bone (looking much like bone meal) is squeezed out of the incision like toothpaste from a tube. Bunion sufferers undergoing this particular technique have been known to be up and about the same day with minimal pain and recovery period. Your feet must be comfortable.

Now let's track back up the body and have a look inside.

## THE HEART

The heart is the toughest organ in the female body—and the least complaining, considering the workload it takes on every minute and hour of the day. Each day your heart beats

100,000 times and pumps 4,300 gallons of blood around the body at a rate of about 1.5 million gallons a year. Men may joke about the "fickle" female heart: in reality, it's a machine of awesome power and endurance. The premenopausal woman, in fact, has a built-in protective shield against cardiovascular disease, due to the unique balance of her female hormones (see the section on heart disease in Chapter 7).

The statistics for heart disease overall do not look too heartening (excuse the pun). First the bad news: cardiovascular, lung, and blood diseases will account for over 1,200,000 deaths a year in the United States—over half of all deaths annually. Now for the good news: in 1983 the death rate for coronary heart disease was 60 percent of what it was in 1963, and among the twenty-six industrialized countries, the United States has the steepest decline in mortality from heart disease in women ages thirty-five to seventy-four. For a woman who is already in her forties, these figures clearly indicate that, as far as heart disease goes, she can look forward to a much longer life span than her mother or grandmother.

But we have to face one thing as we get older: our heart isn't getting any younger. As we pass into the mid-years, there's a tendency for the heart to take on a little extra fat on the exterior walls, especially among those of us who are obese or eat a lot of fatty foods. There are degenerative changes that occur on the inside of the heart due to fat buildup, but these should be of little consequence to a woman in her forties. (For a discussion of coronary artery disease and heart attack, see page 183.)

## THE LUNGS

There should be very little difference between your lungs today and what they were like during your twenties and thirties—provided, that is, you don't smoke. Although the chest wall grows slightly over the years in width and depth, and will continue to do so until you are about sixty, the healthy lung at forty will have very little less volume than when you were younger. This slightly diminished capacity of the lungs is quite natural, because these paired organs do deteriorate, albeit slowly, as we get older.

The decreased lung volume is the result not of the lungs shrinking but of a buildup of residue in the pulmonary tissues. Although they are self-cleaning (for example, coughing is a natural method of bringing up unwanted debris from the lungs; the offending material is coated with mucus to ease its passage through the bronchial tubes), they must put up with a tremendous amount of abuse from pollutants and chemicals in the atmosphere. Their job is to filter out all the garbage we breathe and prevent it from getting into the bloodstream. Over the years, small deposits of residue will build up in pockets in the lungs, thereby robbing us of some of the volume we had in our younger years.

One of the greatest values of regular exercise is that it not only tunes up muscles and strengthens the heart but also conditions the lungs and aids in the cleaning process. The major risk factors for damage to the lungs are smoking, being in a smoky environment (passive smoke inhalation), or living in an industrial area that is constantly threatened with air pollution. Don't think that if you're not a smoker yourself you run no risk of developing lung cancer. Recent research has shown that female nonsmokers who are married to smokers have a significantly higher risk of developing lung disease than do those who are married to nonsmokers.

Respiratory problems are becoming much more frequent than they used to be in women. More people are developing asthma than ever before. If you had hay fever or eczema as a child, it is quite possible that you may experience respiratory spasms or asthma attacks after exposure to viral infection or to some particles (especially dust, pollen, feathers, chemicals, and animal dander) in the air to which you may suddenly develop a sensitivity. Luckily, diagnostic techniques and treatment are much more sophisticated today for sudden respiratory problems. If you notice breathlessness or cough-

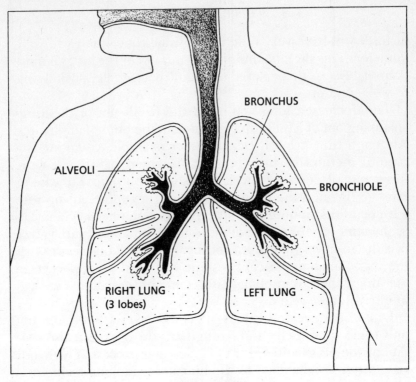

BRONCHUS

ALVEOLI

BRONCHIOLE

RIGHT LUNG
(3 lobes)

LEFT LUNG

## THE LUNGS

This simple diagram illustrates the positioning and components of
the lungs. Lung cancer is on the increase among women. *National
Cancer Institute*

ing during exertion or when breathing cold air, discuss this
with your physician. He will give you a prescription medication to treat the condition and advice on how to prevent it
from happening again. If the problem becomes chronic, I
strongly suggest that you consult an allergy or pulmonary
specialist.

And for those of you who still smoke, the news is getting
worse. When you have smoked for twenty to thirty years, 4
percent of you will get lung cancer. The leading cause of
cancer deaths in women, lung cancer, is up to thirty times
more common in women who smoke. Although it most often
strikes women in their fifties and sixties, we can't predict for

sure when it will arise. Another sad fact is that 14 percent of women who work with asbestos will develop lung cancer (see Chapter 7).

## THE LIVER

The liver, our largest internal organ, is responsible for most of the complicated chemical processes in the body, including control of glucose, manufacture of plasma proteins, lipid (fatty acid) and lipoproteins, and synthesis of bile, which is secreted by the liver into the intestine to digest fats. Vitamins A, $B_{12}$, D, E, and K are stored in the liver, which also creates necessary enzymes from other chemicals and detoxifies drugs and chemicals in the bloodstream, breaking them down into more manageable formulae for excretion. It is the powerhouse industrial plant of the body. Fortunately, it has a very large reserve capacity for work and there is very little alteration of function at your age, unless you have been a habitual consumer of large amounts of alcohol over the years or had liver disease. Otherwise, your liver should be in excellent shape.

Both blood flow to this organ and its size diminish slightly as you approach your forties, but in no way should this interfere with the liver's crucial role in these essential body processes. It is easy to test liver function by performing simple blood tests, and these will be ordered by your physician should a liver problem be suspected. Biopsy of the liver is now a safe procedure (serious complications are less than ½ percent), when it is occasionally necessary to differentiate between liver-disease states.

Cirrhosis of the liver is the end result of scarring by fibrous tissue that surrounds liver cells and damages them by distorting the normal architecture and diminishing the blood supply necessary for normal function. Its most common cause in the Western world is chronic abuse of alcohol, while in underdeveloped countries the cause is usually liver infection with the hepatitis B virus. Liver damage by alcohol is made worse by the malnutrition and vitamin deficiency seen in many chronic alcoholics.

At the age of forty, if you have problems with excessive intake of alcohol, it is not too late to stop poisoning your liver and start following a sensible balanced diet. Many other medical conditions lead to liver problems as secondary complications, such as hemochromatosis, an iron-overload syndrome, and certain connective-tissue diseases.

Cirrhosis is often silent in that the patient has no symptoms and the liver appears to function well. It would seem wise, therefore, to level with your doctor about your use of alcohol so that recommendations may be made for your liver to retain its vital function for as long as possible.

## THE KIDNEYS

Unless you have suffered from a serious kidney infection in recent years, or have been diagnosed as having kidney dysfunction (when the kidneys fail to perform), there really is no reason to think that these two organs are working at anything other than peak efficiency. Like the lungs, the kidneys deteriorate gradually with age, but at forty you should not be experiencing any perceivable difference in functioning from earlier on in your life. Also like the lungs, the kidneys are filter organs: they remove toxins and other unwanted substances from our bodies.

The age-related decline in kidney function is something a doctor must take into account when prescribing certain drugs that are excreted through the kidneys.

## THE DIGESTIVE SYSTEM

At the age of forty, you may be able to make some changes that will prevent problems fifteen or twenty years from now.

Diverticulosis is a condition in which little pockets of the intestinal lining are formed that protrude through the muscle layers of the gut, usually the colon. It is thought to be caused by chronic constipation. A diet low in fiber produces hard stools of small bulk, and years of forcing these stools through your colon results in this condition, though it may not cause symptoms for a long time. As you get older, the pockets may become infected and cause episodes of acute abdominal pain, fever, and even bowel obstruction. Diverticulosis is thus responsible for chronic illness and even intestinal surgery in older individuals.

Chronic constipation also causes hemorrhoids in susceptible women (look to heredity again!), so watch your eating habits and follow a diet high in fiber content. You may save yourself a lot of trouble when you're older (see Chapter 7).

You should also know the risk factors for colon cancer, the third leading cause of cancer deaths in women. You are susceptible if you have had any of the following:

- Inflammatory bowel disease
- History of cancer of the colon or adenoma (benign tumor of the lining of the bowel)
- Familial polyposis, a hereditary disorder of benign large-intestine polyps
- History of breast or gynecological cancer
- Years of diet low in fiber and high in animal fat, especially beef
- Family history of colon cancer in a first-degree relative

Screening for and prevention of this type of cancer should start when you are forty. A rectal examination should be performed after your pelvic examination and your stool checked for microscopic blood. If this should prove positive, then you will need X-ray or endoscopic (visual) examination of your bowel using a proctosigmoidoscope, a flexible tube with a fiber optic lighting system inserted into the rectum. If you are in the high-risk category, especially if you have a family history of bowel cancer, this examination is recommended at intervals, starting at age forty and performed more frequently as you get older. Signs of colon cancer are a change in bowel habits or in caliber of stools; passage of blood, bright red or maroon-colored; and vague abdominal pain (see also page 211).

## THE THYROID

An overactive thyroid gland can cause an array of problems. Known as hyperthyroidism, or Graves' disease, this condition occurs five times more often in women than men and usually develops between the ages of thirty and fifty. You are in the prime age range for thyroid problems to manifest themselves.

The thyroid weighs less than an ounce and is located in the neck next to the windpipe and below the voice box. The cause of hyperthyroidism is still mostly a mystery, although the disorder is thought by many to be an autoimmune disease (when the immune system turns against itself). Symptoms include nervousness, increased activity, undue sweating, increased appetite, insomnia, weight loss, heart palpitations, a decreased tolerance for heat, irregularity of menstrual periods, and excessively oily hair and skin. Physical signs of the condition may include swelling of the thyroid gland and staring, protruding eyes.

In hyperthyroidism the gland, for some unknown reason, starts to pump out an excessive amount of the thyroid hormone. Personality changes may be associated with the condition, especially mood swings, anxiety, irritability, frequent crying jags, and depression. Because of these emotional symptoms, which may be more pronounced than the enlargement of the thyroid gland or other telltale signs, Graves' disease has occasionally been treated initially as a psychiatric disorder. Doctors and mental health professionals need to be vigilant: a simple blood test diagnoses hyperthyroidism and the emotional symptoms subside when the condition is treated properly. Treatment consists of medications that impede the output of thyroid hormone; noninvasive radioactive iodine treatment, which destroys the gland; or surgical removal of part or all of the gland.

Hypothyroidism is exactly the opposite—an underproduction of the thyroid hormone. Here again women are far more susceptible than men. We are four times more likely than men to develop this condition. As you would expect, the symptoms are the opposite of those of an overactive thyroid. They include: swollen, puffy neck and face, sensitivity to cold, dry, scaly skin, excessive menstruation, hair loss, constipation, and intellectual impairment and emotional disturbances, Again, diagnosis is simple and treatment involves thyroid hormone replacement therapy, commonly thyroxine on a daily basis. While treatment may be necessary for life, it is important for a physician to monitor the condition on a regular basis, because the output of thyroid hormone does diminish as we age.

There is also a condition known as hyperparathyroidism that occurs twice as often in women as in men. It is estimated that one out of every thousand routine blood tests will identify an existing condition of hyperparathyroidism. This problem involves overproductive parathyroid glands and an increased production of parathyroid hormone (PTH), which controls how we metabolize calcium in the bone, kidneys, and gastrointestinal tract. In hyperparathyroidism, excess PTH causes increased calcium in the blood and the urine. Because the level of calcium is out of balance, the condition can lead to increased incidence of bone fractures, kidney stones, and muscular weakness. Treatment of hyperparathyroidism aims to control the excessive levels of calcium. The parathyroid glands can be removed, and this proves to be successful in over 90 percent of cases.

So: the answer to "Where am I now?" is as easy as saying "Wherever you want to be!" As set forth in this chapter, being forty doesn't mean that it's time to watch your body going downhill. Quite the opposite, in fact. From what you've just read, it must be patently obvious that this is prime time to change old bad habits and begin a new program to fine-tune that sleek and sporty feminine machine.

# 2

# Forms and Curves

Oh, wouldn't it be wonderful if we were all racehorse slender, pencil-slim, sylphlike, and shaped to order? No, of course not. We'd all look like production-line robots. When you think about the shape you're in, the forms and curves that make up your exterior image, remember one thing: nature comes in infinite variety.

Undoubtedly you've been staring into the mirror for the last few years worrying about those few extra pounds here and there and maybe that inch or so on the waist and buttocks. If you go by what you see in the looking glass every day, there's a good chance you will be disappointed with what you see, for one simple reason. As women, we always tend to perceive the female ideal as being a little more shapely and a lot less heavy than in fact we are. What you actually see in the mirror, however, is not the real you—or at least not as others see you. Because of the reflective image and a mental attitude that perceives our own bodies as plumper than they are, we get an overall distorted picture of our real selves. If you want to prove this to yourself, just find a friend (preferably a close friend for this experiment) you would consider about the same size and shape as you. Then take a tape measure and accurately record each other's measurements from the neck down: upper arms, breasts, waist, buttocks, thighs, calves, and even ankles and feet. Then compare notes. I'll guarantee you one thing: your statistics will turn out much trimmer than those of your friend—if she still *is* your friend after you explain why you're doing this! Actually, she'll probably get a big kick out of it. "Fancy you ever thinking you were my size," she'll probably respond. "You have a much better figure than I do!"

So you see, the image we have of our own bodies is nothing to go by. The old expression about beauty being "in the eyes of the beholder" is perfectly true—yet this time in reverse. It's all a matter of the way we view things, especially our own forms and curves. Whatever shape you're in, it's probably one that you're not happy with, but the big message is that there are those who adore you for it.

## THE SHAPE WE'RE IN

What we should be far more concerned about in our forties is not the visual but the physical shape we're in. And that means everything from muscle tone to fat content. No doubt you will have gained a few extra pounds through your thirties, but that's to be expected. Our metabolic rate has been slowing down, so, in a perfect world—assuming you haven't been doing anything drastically different during the past decade—you will have gained weight. But, unless it is an extraordinary amount, it will probably be perceivable only to yourself. That's because as women, thanks to the estrogen we have coursing around our bodies, we have a natural dispersal and displacement ability. Unlike men, who will take on extra luggage around the waist, we divide it out quite evenly over the lower trunk, hips, buttocks, and thighs. In other words, we can make a little gained weight go a much longer way. You should get another

43

important message from that news: it's not always good to go by what the scale says. What may be a five- or even ten-pound weight gain may, depending on your frame size, go totally unnoticed by those around you. Don't panic when comparing pounds and ounces to your fighting weight in your twenties and thirties.

Take heart: you may indeed be in far better shape than you ever imagined—especially when it comes to weight.

## Weight

There's good news for all women in their forties when assessing their ideal weight. Most women who believe they are "unreasonably" overweight are actually not. And now there are indications that women who are a little overweight are far healthier than those who are either obese or underweight. In Massachusetts, a long-term epidemiological study of women ages forty to sixty-nine discovered that the highest death rate was among the thinnest and the most obese, with the lowest among the broad range of women in the intermediate weight ranges.

For years we have been prisoners of the "ideal" weight scales drawn up by the insurance companies. These scales have traditionally tipped toward leanness. The National Heart, Lung, and Blood Institute reports that standard weight tables produce more stress for Americans who consider themselves overweight than does rising inflation. And the National Institutes of Health recently reported that thin women have a higher mortality rate than do those of average or slightly above average weight. What does all this mean? Well, because of pressure from the medical profession, the Society of Actuaries and the Life Insurance Medical Directors of America have recently revised their "ideal" weight tables in a welcome upward direction.

It's now generally agreed that the old guidelines for "normal weight" among the female population should be increased by as much as ten pounds on average. So check how you shape up on the following revised table:

## Ideal Weight Chart for Females

| | Frame Size | | |
|---|---|---|---|
| | SMALL | MEDIUM | LARGE |
| HEIGHT | | POUNDS | |
| 4'8" | 86–89 | 93–103 | 98–118 |
| 4'9" | 88–99 | 95–106 | 100–121 |
| 4'10" | 90–102 | 97–109 | 102–124 |
| 4'11" | 92–105 | 99–112 | 105–127 |
| 5' | 93–111 | 100–117 | 106–128 |
| 5'1" | 95–117 | 101–122 | 107–130 |
| 5'2" | 100–122 | 104–128 | 109–133 |
| 5'3" | 104–128 | 109–133 | 113–139 |
| 5'4" | 109–133 | 113–139 | 118–144 |
| 5'5" | 113–139 | 118–144 | 122–150 |
| 5'6" | 118–144 | 122–150 | 127–155 |
| 5'7" | 122–150 | 127–155 | 131–161 |
| 5'8" | 127–155 | 131–161 | 136–166 |
| 5'9" | 131–161 | 136–166 | 140–172 |
| 5'10" | 136–166 | 140–172 | 145–177 |
| 5'11" | 140–172 | 145–177 | 149–183 |
| 6' | 145–177 | 149–183 | 154–188 |
| 6'1" | 150–182 | 154–187 | 159–194 |

Find your frame size by measuring the circumference of your dominant wrist (the wrist you write with). Small—less that 6 inches; medium—6–6.5 inches; large—over 6.5 inches.

Height: Always take measurement in stocking feet.

You can easily see from this table that we have much more leeway to play with when it comes to assessing ideal weight for optimal health.

## Fat Flaws

I'm going to give you this one straight from the hip! If nobody ever told you before, now's the time to learn. You cannot remove fat—unless, that is, you are a skilled surgeon. Fat is not something that just disappears. "Oh, no!" you say. "How come my best friend Sheila lost those thirty pounds on the Remarkable Rhubarb, Radish, and Rutabaga Diet?" The truth is that your friend Sheila was able to shrink the fat cells in her body; she never actually got rid of any. When you lose weight through diet, you decrease the size of fat cells but not the number. And here's the unpleasant part: you're stuck with the number of fat cells you presently have. The number of cells you've accumulated was actually determined when you were in infancy and later around the time of puberty. If you were a plump youngster and a chubby adolescent, chances are you'll always gravitate back to this shape throughout the rest of your life. This is why so many women find it so hard to lose those extra pounds and keep them off; they've actually been preprogrammed earlier in life to be the shape they're in. I've had patients come to me who have been on diets that supply fewer than eight hundred or nine hundred calories a day (a low level that I'm extremely uncomfortable with, even over the short term) and they complain of losing weight at an agonizingly slow rate. I have to be brutally honest: "I'm sorry. Maybe you're just not biologically cut out to be skinny," . . . and I emphasize the "skinny." As a doctor, I'm extremely concerned about obesity: since it's one of the biggest health problems we face in this country, I'm the first to advise any overweight person to shed a few pounds. But I have to be honest: if a woman is not overweight to the extent that it impinges on her

46

good health, I'll tell her to luxuriate in her bountiful figure because that's the way Mother Nature intended her to be.

However, there is such a thing as having a relatively moderate number of fat cells yet still being too plump. This is a much easier problem to overcome, because you were not predestined to be fat. Possibly your life-style, diet, and sedentary habits have made you that way. Dieting and exercise are sure to help, and if you don't return to bad old habits, you're likely to keep your new form and curves.

Also, please don't be taken in by all the gimmicks out there on the market to remove "women's worst enemy," cellulite. People who manufacture those rubber sweatpants and bizarre "cellulite-removing" machines with belts that pound away at your body would just love you to think that cellulite is some magically dissolvable substance, when in reality it is nothing more than groups of regular fat cells that have clumped together in pockets, probably due to reduced muscle and skin tone. They have that rippled or cobbled feel because of their structure and because the skin may have lost some of the elasticity that would otherwise help disguise these cells.

You should treat cellulite exactly the same as you would other layers of fat on the body. Pummeling and pounding one particular spot will not remove fat from that area. Only progressive exercise combined with a reduced caloric intake will help you lose fat—and it will be an *overall* process, not selective to one spot. Bear in mind that when total fat content is reduced, cellulite will be less noticeable. (See Chapter 3, on the cosmetics of skin.)

There is, however, another option—slicing or suctioning away the fat. The surgeon's scalpel or "vacuum cleaner" is usually the last resort for dispensing with unwanted fat. I'm not against these methods, but you should really try all your other weight-loss options first. Having said that, I can report that many women are highly delighted with their buttock and breast lifts, tummy tucks, and other antigravity saviors. Modern cosmetic surgery is a fine art, and mostly risk-free today.

If you feel you need to be sculptured by the scalpel, make sure you know what you're getting into and go for it—provided you can afford the price tag. Mostly you pay for what you get (see charts on pages 72–73).

Much of the way you appear at forty has less to do with you than with your genetic destiny.

## A Matter of How the Genes Fit

No doubt you've heard the male expression "If you want to see what she'll be like twenty years from now, take a good look at her mother!" To a degree this is true. If you have followed approximately the same life-style and steered a similar course as your mother or grandmother, and provided they have not been affected by disease states, glandular obesity, or hormonal problems, you can expect to be pretty much in the same shape when you hit their age. If you have daughters, they can be looking at you today as a role model for their forties. Heredity is a strong determinant of your physical makeup. And in this regard, don't forget to take Dad into account as well. While you are female and think you might take after only your mother, there may be some genetic traits you received from your father.

I have two grown daughters who are totally different from each other in shape and build. One takes more after her father: she has a robust build, a short neck, large rib cage, wide hips, and strong thighs and calves. My other daughter has a long neck, a narrow rib cage and a smaller frame and is considerably taller. So, when you want to assess the shape of things to come, take a good look at the family tree and decide which parent you take after most.

My build has always leaned toward strength. I've never had a slender frame, although my legs were always slender and shapely, with slim ankles. But I have a large rib cage, less of an indention at the waist and narrower than normal hips (not the most ideal for childbearing, I might add). I've always had

48

tremendously strong hands and powerful wrists—an absolute godsend when it comes to delivering babies! At times, like any other woman, I've rebelled against my figure, wishing it was a little more sylphlike. But there have been other times when I've been thankful for the strength and endurance my body has given me: during times like pregnancy and rearing my children or when endless hours in labor wards and maternity units could have taken their toll.

## PREGNANCY AND SHAPE

While we're on the subject, I'd like to make a few remarks about my own pregnancies. You may find them useful. As I mentioned, my narrow hips are not ideal for childbirth, yet I gave birth to two rather large girls, the first nine pounds four ounces, the second nine pounds fourteen ounces. Both had to be born by C-section. My middle baby, a boy, weighed in at seven pounds four ounces, and actually gave me more trouble than the girls. I was in bed for six months while I carried him. There was no ultrasound then to diagnose the problem: the long weeks lying in bed hoping the baby would be normal were quickly forgotten when our lively son was born. You just can't account sometimes for Mother Nature throwing you a curve.

As far as physical shape goes, there really shouldn't be too much difference from when you were in your teens and twenties. Surprised? You shouldn't be if you've taken good care of your body. There are, however, two things that may have gotten a little larger from childbirth—your feet. Heavier pregnancies tend to put more strain on the feet, and they can spread and flatten a little. Since I had my children my shoe size went up one and one-half sizes.

On the whole, apart from a little extra weight gain during your thirties and forties, you should expect to be pretty much in the same shape as you were a decade or so ago.

# BLOATING

This is a common problem we females face—but mostly one of vanity and of little or no medical concern. Bloating is usually only a matter of water retention. The more fluid that enters the cells of our deeper skin layers, the more we tend to puff up. It may even be more apparent in our forties as we lose a little elasticity and tone in our skin.

Bloating typically occurs just before our periods and is usually bothersome only from a cosmetic point of view, when we try to wriggle into that tightest pair of jeans. Therefore, doesn't it make sense to have a few clothes on the side that are a little less than form-fitting?

Fluid retention and constant bloating should be taken seriously, however, as it may be an indication of high blood pressure. Many women who suffer from high blood pressure are put on diuretics, drugs that dispel fluid retention. It's not unusual for a woman to lose a few pounds once she is on a course of diuretics—a side effect many of us don't mind one bit!

# EXERCISE

When you start an exercise program, you have to kick one addiction—the scale habit. Don't keep jumping on the scale every day and expecting to see weight loss. In fact, even though you're burning off fat, you're building muscle tissue. So, what's the difference? A big one: muscle weighs more than fat. You may actually *gain* a few pounds at the beginning of a fitness and exercise program while trimming off a few inches at the same time. Most of the fat in your body is located under your skin and over the muscles. Firming up the muscles will give you a slimmer appearance. So the best advice I can give is to watch the tape measure instead of the scale.

What's the best course of exercise for you? Quite frankly,

whatever appeals to you as an individual. Some women will thrive on racquetball or squash, while others may find it too arduous or competitive. Two or three leisurely games of tennis a week may be more your speed. Bicycling, walking, or running are all grand forms of exercise. What really matters most is that you are making the effort to do some form of exercise. Even a little, if you haven't already been doing any, is worth its weight loss in gold.

There are about 20 million women out there jumping, bopping, and grinding to music for exercise. Aerobic dancing has really caught on, and most women, once they get over the initial aches and pains, find it one of the most inexpensive and pleasurable forms of exercise. I would highly recommend it for the body at forty.

Although there is no physiological reason why a woman in her forties should not be able to undertake the exercise regimen of a twenty-year-old, the chances are that what with having babies, raising children, and keeping a home—not to mention the demands of a job or career—it's more than likely that exercise has not been a permanent part of your life-style. It's for this reason that plunging headlong into a heavy-duty program is not a good idea. If you want to gravitate to this later, fine—but start with an aerobics course first to tone up those muscles and stretch out the ligaments and tendons.

By now you should have a good overall idea of your body as far as its forms and curves go.

# 3

# Our Cosmetic Selves

No other part of our body plays a more important social and esthetic role than our largest organ—the skin. It instantly reflects our femininity, our health, and our personality. And now that we've reached forty, it's starting to show our age, too! Decades of ultraviolet rays, cosmetics, harsh cleansers, and even birth-control pills are taking their toll. Suddenly, age spots are beginning to appear on our wrists, and facial wrinkles are getting tougher to cover up.

Thank goodness science isn't leaving us out in the cold, though. Exciting breakthroughs allow us to turn the clock back and, in a way, give our skin a second childhood.

## OUR CHANGING SKIN

Dermatologists are always telling us that most skin problems could be prevented by avoiding harmful conditions in the environment. Unfortunately, when we're young—with soft, supple, radiant skin—such advice falls on deaf ears. "How could my skin ever become tough and wrinkled? That happens only to old people." Remember making those statements? I certainly do. Alas, as most of us can now attest, the day of the first wrinkle arrives long before old age.

But first, a quick lesson about this most sensitive organ of ours:

The outer layer of skin, the epidermis, grows constantly and renews itself every thirty days to replace the dead cells we are constantly shedding. Conservatively speaking, you've already had almost five hundred "skin lifts" during your lifetime. The epidermis acts as a two-way barrier to prevent body fluids from leaking out and external fluids, like bath water, from seeping in. If it wasn't for this tough outer layer, we'd soak up water like a sponge every time we went into the shower or out for a swim! Beneath the epidermis is the dermis, a strong supportive structure of fibrous tissue, glands, nerves, and blood vessels. It's interwoven with millions of elastic fibers that act like Spandex clothing—preventing puckering at certain sites, such as the elbows and knees, that constantly stretch and bend. Below the dermis lies a layer of fat that insulates the inner body against excessive heat or cold.

And it's this subcutaneous fat that's to blame for the most obvious skin changes that have started to appear now that we're in our forties.

## WRINKLES

Don't you just hate it when someone points out that our lives are now probably more than half over? Yet, even though our best years are yet to come and we feel great, something's happening just below the surface of our skin that is going to make us quickly realize we're definitely changing.

That layer of fat that cushions the surface skin is slowly being absorbed by the body. And because the elastic fibers in the dermis are also breaking down, the external skin doesn't have the capability to shrink at the same rate. Result: the skin tends to collapse and become enfolded, forming wrinkles. The effect may be likened to that of a balloon: when it's been blown up for a while, the rubber surface adjusts in size to the cushion of air within. But release some of that cushion and the surface becomes wrinkled. The more cushion that's taken away, the more pronounced the wrinkles.

But why are some people graced with smooth, wrinkle-free skin well into their forties and beyond? It's not just a matter of good looks and good luck. Certainly heredity does make a difference: the darker and thicker our skin, the less visibly we'll age. But other factors are far more significant. The secret to youthful-looking skin at our age is continuous preventive care. Fortunately, even once the damage is done, new advances in skin care can help rejuvenate almost anyone's face and body.

## The Sun Factor

The skin's biggest enemy isn't time; it's repeated exposure to the sun. The radiation that gives us that glowing tan also hastens damage to the skin. Yet, no matter how many times we're told, we American women just can't help "going for the burn." One glance along the beaches of this country from coast to coast in the summertime reveals millions of fair-skinned people soaking up the sun's rays. And during the winter months, you'll find them in tanning parlors, getting another dose of ultraviolet radiation. Well, what may look and feel good at age twenty doesn't look and feel so good at our age. A well-tanned skin on an older woman often looks dry and wrinkled, and is sun-damaged and cancer-prone.

Sunscreens seem the only effective answer at the moment. Not only do they dramatically reduce the risk of further skin damage, they also protect us against skin cancer, which, during the next ten years, will strike more than 5 million Americans. You and I are now entering the high-risk age for this disease. The statistics are grim. Not only does skin cancer kill eight thousand Americans a year, it also leaves thousands more disfigured with scars, following removal of malignant growths affecting the nose, eyes, lips, and ears.[1]

Surgery is the method of treatment in 90 percent of cases, although researchers are testing other techniques, including heating and freezing tumors. Almost 20 percent of skin cancers are so advanced that when patients finally decide to seek medical help they're inoperable. That's where laser therapy may hold the key. University of Cincinnati researchers recently reported exciting results using lasers to treat terminally ill skin-cancer patients. They've treated all three forms—melanoma (the most deadly type), squamous cell, and basal cell—and in every patient, the tumor vanished. The patients are being closely monitored to see if there's any recurrence, but so far the technique is looking good.

As with other forms of cancer, early detection dramatically improves your chance for a cure. The American Cancer Society urges us to be on the lookout for any change in the size or color of a mole or other darkly pigmented growth or spot. Scaliness, oozing, bleeding, or the sudden appearance of a bump or nodule are other signs of cancer developing. Those of us with a fair complexion are at even higher risk, so be on your guard. It's never too late to start protecting yourself.

## Sunscreens

They're not all alike. The effectiveness of sunscreens is denoted by a number called the sun protective factor (SPF). Generally, the SPF ranges from 2 to 15, with 15 offering the most protection. There are three different types of chemical sunscreens commercially available: para-aminobenzoic acid (PABA) or PABA-derivative sunscreens; non-PABA sunscreens; and combination sunscreens. Most sunscreens contain PABA or PABA derivatives. Read the label! The American Cancer Society strongly recommends that we use sunscreens containing PABA because they've been shown to protect against sun damage significantly while still allowing us to tan, if we wish. It has been determined that, for the best protection, we should apply a screen at least thirty minutes before lying out in the sun. This gives it time to bind to the cells of the skin.

University of California scientists conducted an extensive investigation into skin damage from the sun and concluded that all of us should apply a sunscreen with a 15 SPF during exposure to intense ultraviolet radiation. For most areas of the United States, this means from 10:00 A.M. to 2:00 P.M., March through October, or throughout the year in snow-covered, high-altitude regions or on beaches or when sailing or waterskiing. Those of us with fair skin should wear a sunscreen especially on the face if planning to be in the sun for more than an hour in summertime. Interestingly, the California researchers also found that the ability to tan is genetically determined. No matter how hard you try, if you've got a fair complexion, all you'll achieve is irreversible skin damage. And no matter what it says on the bottle, no lotion can promote or accelerate tanning. Those "fast-tan" products stain the superficial layer of the skin but do not promote the formation of tannin by the body cells, which is what actually creates the darkening of the skin.

## Getting the Wrinkles Out

Our faces have become a multi-billion-dollar business. Everywhere you look, there are new creams, new oils, new surgical techniques—all aimed at giving us a shot at youth again. Of course, there are many admirable women our age who consider wrinkles to be a natural, distinguished sign of aging that marks the face with character. But most of us would love to get rid of them! Hence the boom in cosmetic surgery.

*Collagen implants.* These are now commonly used to reduce the size of wrinkles and age lines. It is a very effective technique, particularly where the lines are deep. Collagen is a natural component of skin, bone, and other tissues. The implants are processed from collagen in cowhide into a form that's compatible with human tissue. The soft, gel-like substance provides a miniature face-lift. It's laced with an anesthetic and implanted under the skin with fine-gauged needles. There it converts into a latticework of collagen fibers, much as individual threads combine to form a piece of cloth. This well-woven mesh becomes the base for new tissue to grow and multiply. Two to six treatments are usually necessary to achieve the desired results.

*Chemical peels.* These will remove tiny wrinkles that are now beginning to appear around our lips and eyes. Physicians developed this procedure after noticing that faces that had healed after moderately severe burns appeared more youthful. The doctor applies a chemical called phenol with a cotton-tip applicator and tapes the treated area. When properly applied, the chemical produces a superficial burn. After forty-eight hours, the physician removes the tape and dries the wound with a water-absorbing powder that encourages a scab to form. The scab falls off in five to seven days, leaving red, dry skin that must be regularly soaked and lubricated with vegetable oil or Vitamin A and D ointment. Voila! As the face heals, skin grows back—*without* the wrinkles. There's some pain attached to the procedure, and the treated areas are unsightly for some days, but no one can deny that the results are remarkable.

*Dermabrasion.* This is another way to erase small facial wrinkles. A machine called an abrator mechanically removes a portion of the top layer of skin. It's rather like sandpapering the rough spots off a piece of wood. Often, people tolerate mechanical abrasion with less pain than they do the chemical peel and the end results are about the same: the skin usually remains wrinkle-free for five years or more.

*Silicone injections.* You've probably heard about silicone only in relation to breasts. Now it's a great new alternative for your skin. Silicone injections help replace that fatty tissue that's absorbed as we get older. However, this technique is usually reserved not for fine wrinkles but for those deep furrows that occur on the forehead and between the eyes.

**Fat-autograft.** One of the most exciting new developments is the fat-autograft technique, in which live fat cells are sucked out of one part of the body and used to fill in undesirable facial lines. It's so simple I'm amazed it wasn't discovered years ago. Using a needle and suction device, the plastic surgeon simply sucks fat cells from any available area of the body—most often the buttocks, hips, or tummy—and injects them beneath the wrinkles and facial lines to eliminate the skin fold. Fat-cell grafts have the advantage of being an excellent filling substance because they're simply replacing what was there before. And, of course, there's no risk of rejection or allergy, as it's the patient's own tissue. The results are likely to be long-lasting, too: it's a living substance that continues to stay alive and reproduce.

New York plastic surgeon Lawrence Reed, a pioneer of the technique, reports: "It may well be the most ideal substance for filling soft-tissue defects anyplace on the body and its lasting effectiveness spans several years."

## AGE SPOTS AND OTHER BLEMISHES

In Grandma's day they were called liver spots—those flat, circular patches of brown pigment that are now beginning to appear on the backs of our hands, face, and neck. That was, perhaps, a kinder way of describing what today are referred to as age spots. And our driving habits are probably to blame. Yes, you heard me right!

In the United States, where we drive on the right, more people develop age spots on their left arms and hands than on their right. Conversely, in countries where people drive on the left, as in England and Australia, the pattern is reversed. The reason: sun exposure. When the weather's fine, we all tend to drive with one arm resting on the sill of an open window, so that arm gets more sun than the other. And as sunlight causes age spots, up they pop when we get to our age. Thus, avoiding overexposure to the sun by applying a sunscreen with an SPF of 15 is a surefire way to prevent these spots.

Tan or brown crusty growths, called seborrheic keratoses, can appear just about anywhere and are common at our age, too. But there are techniques available to either remove or reduce the visibility of such blemishes. A dermatologic surgeon has a variety of tools at his disposal; which technique he or she uses depends on the type, size, and location of the growth.

*Cryosurgery.* Freckles and surface keratoses are literally frozen to death when liquid nitrogen is applied directly to them.

*Electrosurgery.* Small blemishes, including broken capillaries, are painlessly burned away with a fine-tipped instrument that zaps them with an electric current.

*Chemoexcoriation.* Brown spots are eradicated by the application of a diluted acid.

*Skin-punch excision.* A circular punch just large enough to fit around a mole or other similar growth punctures the skin and removes the offending blemish. The wound is sutured or allowed to heal naturally. Scarring is minimal and usually doesn't show.

*Shave excision.* Superficial growths are shaved off, using a small, sharp blade.

*Laser surgery.* A small, directed laser beam vaporizes the blemish.

Many of you may have seen or heard of over-the-counter bleaching creams. Take my tip, they're practically useless. If they work at all, it's very slowly, and over the months, the money spent on creams can easily exceed the cost of seeing a dermatologist who can clear up the condition with immediate treatment. If you insist on using a nonprescription cream, be sure to get one that contains a sunscreen. If you don't and you go outside, sunlight can actually make the spots worse!

Another common problem at our age is skin tags—tiny, loose flaps of skin attached to the neck, armpit, groin, and around the eyes. Some people grow dozens of them and are extremely disturbed by them. They needn't be: these are among the simplest and safest growths to remove. Snipping them off with surgical scissors causes little pain, minimal bleeding, and no scarring if done correctly. The treated areas may be a bit tender for a while, but if you avoid harsh scrubbing and, in the case of the eyes, makeup, you'll be better than new in a few days.

We're now at the prime age for development of another annoying female skin disorder—acne rosacea. This facial blemish typically affects the nose or the blush area of the cheeks. Later it can spread to the chin and center of the forehead. The skin turns red and surface blood vessels become permanently dilated. It's usually accompanied by acne-type eruptions.

While there's apparently no genetic basis for it, you'll often find that more than one family member will have it at the same time. The condition is most common in fair-skinned, blue-eyed women of northern-European descent. Unlike acne, it does not involve blackheads or overactive oil glands, and while the cause is unknown, sunlight exposure, alcohol, spices, and hot foods commonly aggravate the flushed appearance. Many people find that their face becomes a mass of red blotches after washing down a four-alarm chili with a few glasses of wine. I have to tell them to blame rosacea and not the piquancy of the food.

A definite cure is yet to be found, but often the acnelike symptoms can be controlled by the same treatments used against common acne. Low doses of antibiotics, such as tetracycline or erythromycin, can be very helpful. If they're not, I sometimes prescribe a new Vitamin-A derivative, isotretinoin. Nothing seems to relieve the red color of the skin, however, although argon-laser therapy will effectively destroy any permanently dilated blood vessels. The laser leaves only minimal scarring, compared with cauterizing with an electrically heated instrument.

# HAIR

Does your husband or boyfriend have wavy hair . . . hair that's *waving good-bye?* I know it's an old pun, but have you ever wondered if the same could happen to you? It is a fact that millions of women will be plagued by thinning hair, and, unfortunately, we're now at a prime age for it to start to happen.

It occurs for a variety of reasons, the most common of which is changes in our hormone balance at the approach of menopause. But other disorders that tend to strike after the age of forty can trigger significant thinning: iron deficiency, diabetes, ovarian cysts, and thyroid problems. Even stress and psychological trauma can cause hair loss.

If you seem to be losing more than usual, it's not necessarily cause for alarm. There's a chance the hair will come back. Whatever you do, don't work yourself up into a lather: anxiety tends to aggravate hair loss. Relax—there are simple steps you can take to minimize the problem:

- Don't overuse straighteners, blow dryers, and curling irons.
- Avoid perms and bleaches.
- Eat a well-balanced diet.
- Consider a thorough medical checkup.
- Wash your hair daily.
- Don't sleep in rollers.
- Don't pull your hair back tightly in a bun or ponytail.

## Bald Facts

Common male-pattern baldness also strikes women around menopause. It's switched on by the male hormone androgen, which we all have in our bodies to some degree. As our female hormones diminish, androgen can begin to have an effect on

61

our hairline. However, help is on the horizon for this type of hair loss.

Researchers are discovering that certain drugs that inhibit androgen have a positive effect on the hair. For example, a side effect of the blood-pressure drug minoxidil is a coarsening and thickening of the hair. Dermatologists at the University of Illinois have made a lotion from this drug for topical application to the scalp and trials are in progress to see if hair growth will be regenerated. Use of this drug for male-pattern baldness and alopecia areata (lack of hair growing on the scalp) is still considered investigational.[2] Other drugs showing promise in curbing baldness include Aldactone, an antihypertension drug, Tagamet, an antiulcer drug, and cortisone medications.

However, none of us has to feel self-conscious about hair loss until a major breakthrough is announced. The simplest and quickest solution is to wear a hairpiece.

## Hairpieces, Weaving, and Transplants

A good hairpiece is made by lacing individual hairs, synthetic or real, through a piece of mesh. It's held in place by double-faced surgical tape. Hairpieces range in price from $400 to $1,000. There are disadvantages, however. You can't sleep in them and they need cleaning every few weeks. Also, hairpieces may need replacing every year. And removing the tape can be pretty painful. If you want to wear a hairpiece all the time, hair weaving may be the answer.

For between $500 and $1,500, the piece is sewn to your remaining hair with fine nylon thread. It can be trimmed and styled and worn when sleeping or swimming. But care must be taken to dry the hair thoroughly after shampooing, to prevent bacteria from growing beneath the mesh. And because the hairpiece can shift as your natural hair grows, you'll likely need to return for a tightening every six to eight weeks.

A hair transplant is the only permanent method of covering

hair loss. Under a local anesthetic, circles of skin about the size of a pencil eraser are taken from those parts of the head where healthy hair still grows. These plugs are then grafted into holes cut into the thinning areas. About three hundred plugs, each with up to twenty hairs, are usually needed for minimum coverage. Hair transplants provide results that last a lifetime, and while it's expensive—$2,000 to $5,000—it's a one-time cost.

One type of hair loss is both unpredictable and mysterious. It's called alopecia areata and it's estimated that more than 2 million men, women, and children suffer some form of the disorder. Alopecia areata can take one of three forms: a mild case, in which some hair is lost in small circular patches, the loss of all or most of the scalp hair, or the loss of all body hair. Although stress was once thought to be a factor in the onset of the condition, that theory is no longer accepted.

The problem lies in the body's immune system, which becomes supersensitive and goes haywire in otherwise healthy people. Antibodies destroy hair growth, but the hair follicles themselves remain healthy. For that reason, there are many cases of spontaneous regrowth of hair once the body stops fighting itself, sometimes after months, sometimes after ten years or more.

There's no cure for the condition, but there are treatments that are relatively effective. If it is caught early, injecting cortisone into the bald patches sometimes induces hair regrowth. This and another drug, anthralin—a topical ointment used to treat psoriasis—are effective for those who have mild cases. Minoxidil has shown promising results, too. Most debilitating for those with acute cases of alopecia areata is having to deal with the stigma of baldness in a society that looks upon hair as a mark of attractiveness. Women with the condition find it especially difficult to cope. The National Alopecia Areata Foundation has been formed to help people with hair loss through the trauma. It publishes a monthly newsletter and organizes support groups.[3]

# When Too Much Hair's the Problem

Excessive hair growth is a source of annoyance and embarrassment to many women our age. Usually, however, it's no more than a cosmetic problem, although in some cases unwanted hair can be a symptom of a medical condition—usually an endocrine-gland abnormality in which the body starts producing an excessive amount of androgen, the male hormone.

A small amount of androgen is normally produced by the ovaries and adrenal glands in all women and does not affect hair growth. But when too much is present, the result is hirsutism—hair on the chin, upper lip, breasts, abdomen, and other "wrong places." The most common medical cause of androgen overproduction is polycystic ovarian disease, not uncommon at our age. It's usually accompanied by irregular menstruation and, often, infertility.

Sometimes the source of the problem is an ovarian or adrenal tumor. The best means of determining the cause of hirsutism is a test that measures the levels of androgen in the blood. A high level indicates that the problem may be medical and that further tests are needed. Obesity can also stimulate androgen production. If hormone levels are normal and menstruation is regular, the problem is most likely genetic in origin. This is most often seen in women of Mediterranean descent, who tend to be hairier than women of other European origins. Heredity is a strong factor; a woman whose family is hirsute will probably have a higher than average amount of facial and body hair.

Unwanted hair cannot be considered solely a cosmetic problem until a doctor has ruled out the possibility of illness or an underlying disease state. A medical verdict is particularly important when the condition appears or worsens suddenly. If the cause is not a medical condition, one effective treatment is to take an oral contraceptive containing the female hormones estrogen and progesterone, which suppress androgen production.

# Facial Hair

Most of us can't tolerate conspicuous facial hair and we'll try almost anything to get rid of it. Bleaching the hair is often a satisfactory method, especially for "peach fuzz." Painless, safe, and inexpensive, bleaching does not remove the hair, but it has the advantage of making it less noticeable.

Shaving is certainly the easiest, cheapest, and most common way to remove hair, but many women don't like the implication of masculinity in shaving facial hair. Another reason women don't shave their faces is the deep-rooted belief that it causes hair to grow faster and coarser. This is a myth! Despite what many people believe, shaving doesn't increase the rate of hair growth or make it more coarse. It's just another old wives' tale. Real drawbacks to shaving are that it is easy to cut yourself and the new hair is rather stubbly. In addition, shaving offers no permanent solution.

Some of the popular alternatives to shaving include tweezing and waxing. Both techniques have the advantages of speed, no risk of drawing blood, and the removal of nearly the entire hair shaft. The interval between treatment is much longer than with shaving simply because the shaft is removed. However, tweezing and waxing are painful and must be repeated regularly. So what's left?

Well, there's electrolysis. This process removes the hair permanently by destroying the base of individual follicles with a spark of electricity delivered through a very tiny needle under magnification. It's time-consuming and costly, but if performed by a qualified hypertrichologist, the results are excellent. Scarring is minimal with the latest techniques, and the discomfort is only momentary. Most women are so thrilled with their appearance after treatment that they wish they had done it years ago. Electrolysis is usually done weekly or bi-weekly to begin with, but when the situation is under control, a touch-up treatment every few months will keep you looking your best. Make sure your electrologist is properly certified in your state and is recommended by your doctor or friends who have had treatments. I have seen women after electrolysis feel enormously increased confidence in their appearance which has reflected favorably on their personality and social lives.

Chemical depilatories are now gaining acceptance again, even though they've been around since Roman times. Depilatory creams dissolve the unwanted hair so it can simply be wiped off with a washcloth. A thick layer is applied to the skin and left there for between five and fifteen minutes, depending on the formulation. When it's removed, the hair is removed with it. A moisturizer should be applied afterward to suppress any irritation. It will usually be several days before any growth is visible again, and the new hair will not have the stubbly feel of shaven hair. Depilatories are a simple way to keep unwanted hair at bay, especially on the legs and in the armpits. But, while they're considered safe, adverse side effects may occasionally occur. Both the fragrances and the degree of alkalinity in certain preparations can cause a contact dermatitis if they are left on the skin too long. For these reasons, a test sample of the product should be placed on the inner part of the wrist for twenty minutes prior to use. If no irritation occurs, it's safe to use on the face.

## HANDS

Years of hot water, harsh detergents, cleansers, and other abrasive elements have taken their toll on our hands and nails. But there are steps we can all take to alleviate, if not remedy, the problem. Red, rough hands are a common complaint among women our age. Causes are many and include contact dermatitis, eczema, psoriasis, fungus or bacterial infections or allergies.

Detergents and other irritants tend to strip away the surface oils and undermine the skin's capacity to retain water. Moisture within the outer layers of skin is what helps to keep it feeling smooth and soft. Water also helps to make it less susceptible to rashes and itching.

Taking good care of your hands involves avoiding irritants and allergens, putting water back into the skin, and sealing it with a cream or oil. Usually, over-the-counter creams rubbed on damp skin can effectively restore moisture and clear up most problems. Sometimes, however, rashes may be stubborn enough to warrant medication; they usually respond to cortisone creams and tar lotions.

## Protection

Protecting hands on a continual basis involves wearing dermal gloves made of thin white cotton when handling dry, irritating substances; cotton-lined rubber gloves when handling wet or moist ones. Avoid direct contact with irritants whenever possible. Ideally, your hands shouldn't stay in gloves longer than thirty minutes at a time, as perspiration can aggravate dermatitis. When your hands must be immersed in water for household chores, sprinkling powder inside your cotton gloves and then slipping a pair of rubber gloves over them cuts down on excess moisture from sweating. If water seeps into your rubber gloves over the cuffs, exchange the cotton ones immediately for a fresh pair.

If wet work cannot be avoided, try to do it all at once, rather than repeatedly putting your hands in and out of water. After you finish, soak your hands in clean, cool water for about five minutes; then rub a cortisone or hand cream into the wet skin. Pat dry and reapply the cream. For sensitive skin, the best cleansers are mild soaps or soap substitutes, such as Dove, Phase III, Alpha Keri, Lowila, Basis, Purpose, Neutrogena, Oilatum, and Kauma. Avoid very hot water, even with gloves on, and don't apply excessive pressure or rub hands vigorously. After your hands get back to normal, continue applying cortisone cream but gradually decrease applications over the next two to four weeks.

# NAILS

Having attractive, healthy, durable nails at our age is no great secret. Basically, it involves proper care and cleansing, protecting hands from harsh chemicals, and a sensible approach to one of our most popular habits—polishing.

The nail consists of dead protein. The only living portion, the matrix, from which new tissue grows, is located under the base. The visible tip of this matrix is the light-shaded, moon-shaped crescent that's especially obvious on the thumb and the big toe. The cuticle is simply a collection of discarded cells and acts as a protective frame that seals skin to the nail and keeps foreign particles out. Clear and translucent, the nail rests on top of a foundation called the nail bed, whose pinkish-red color results from the blood vessels coursing through it.

Normally, nails grow at a rate of about one-half to one millimeter a week. It takes about five months to grow a new nail from scratch, though a hyperactive thyroid can accelerate the pace.

## Polishing

Contrary to what many women think, nail polish does not make nails stronger or less breakable. In fact, continual application and removal has just the opposite effect. Ingredients in both polish and removers—such as dyes, solvents, plasticizers, hardeners, and gloss enhancers—can cause allergic reactions or irritation around the nail and also, eventually, weaken its surface, making it vulnerable to splintering and breakage. While nail tissue will replace itself in time, it often can't do so fast enough to offset the damage.

If you must polish, do it no more than once a week. To remove polish, soak your nails in warm olive oil for a few minutes; then take it off with a very sparse amount of oil-based remover. Try to keep your nails away from paint thinners, insecticides, kerosene, laundry detergents, grease, clay, cutting oils, degreasers, and harsh soaps. Beware of artificial nails, too, especially those containing acrylics or acrylic monomers (read the label!). Such ingredients may result in rashes around the cuticle or swelling of the nail bed, which is frequently mistaken for a stubborn fungus infection.

## Cuticles

Removing cuticles can lead to bleeding and infection, and clipping cuticles carelessly sometimes results in hangnails. It's better to soak your nails first in a mild, soapy solution, then push the cuticles back with a Q-tip. To keep skin moist and avoid hangnails, apply olive oil, moisturizing cream, or pure lanolin, then pat dry before manicuring. Inflamed cuticles can be caused by a yeast or staph infection, and nail separation from its bed can be caused by two types of fungi—warts and other benign tumors growing under the nail. Your dermatologist can clear up these problems.

## Blemishes

Pitting, ridging, stippling, or a gridlike pattern on the nails is often associated with a condition called alopecia areata, which causes circular patches of baldness in men and women (see p. 63). And pigmented stripes, which can result from trauma or internal bleeding, can also be a sign of skin cancer. Sometimes, changes in the texture and color of the nails can signal an internal infection or underlying disease—such as anemia, thyroid disorders, tumors, diabetes, or lung disease—or be a side effect of certain drugs, such as antibiotics. So you see, a great-looking set of nails isn't out of reach. Just watch your general health so they get all the nutrients they need, and practice proper grooming and protection.

# THE BODY WHOLE

There comes a time in most of our lives when we stand in front of the mirror and wish we could rearrange what we see. Take that bit there and insert it over here; throw away that bulge altogether and tuck that piece in! The period of self-criticism and wishful thinking usually begins right about now. Standing there naked, we can't help noticing that things are not quite what they used to be!

But no need to despair: every day, it seems, some innovation in plastic surgery is being announced. Surgeons are using increasingly sophisticated techniques and developing new medical instruments and materials to expand their expertise in cosmetic operations. A burgeoning demand from women our age is constantly bringing prices within the reach of millions more.

Check the list from the American Academy of Facial, Plastic and Reconstructive Surgery on pages 72 and 73.

As you can see, plastic surgery is no longer reserved for the rich and famous. It's now within the reach of you and me, too. But let's take a closer look at some of the major advances that have recently been reported.

## Body Fat

Perhaps the most dramatic innovation is fat-suction surgery, technically called suction lipectomy. This involves inserting a needle beneath the skin of an area you'd like slimmed down and using a suction device to withdraw some of the fat cells. But it's not for everybody. According to the cosmetic experts, it's for those of us with "abnormal fat distribution"—fatty deposits out of proportion to the rest of the body, fat that resists even dedicated dieting. I suspect every woman over forty would claim to fall into that category!

Suction lipectomy works best when the skin is elastic enough to spring back after the fat is removed. For baggier, less resilient skin, the surgeon may have to remove the excess, which means longer excision lines and extra scars. Note, too, that the surgery will not fix textural skin problems, such as cellulite. Although cellulite is fatty tissue, the cottage-cheese appearance is due to the fibers that bind the fat. So, while the fat can be removed, the skin texture will remain the same. (More about cellulite later.)

"Saddlebag" thighs, the abdomen, hips, buttocks, and knees are the most suitable areas for this type of surgery. Ankles and arms can be suctioned on some patients, depending on the delicacy and amount of excess skin that would need to be removed.

Usually, the price of suction-lipectomy surgery ranges from $1,000 to $3,000, but it can be more, depending on the length and complexity of the operation and where you live (prices vary with location). And, as it's considered elective surgery, most insurance plans won't cover it.[4]

Complications from this surgery are rare. When they have occurred, they've been one or more of the following:

- *Contour irregularities.* When too much fat is removed or when fat is removed unevenly, a wavy, lumpy look can result.
- *Shock.* If excessive fat is suctioned, there can be significant fluid loss, leading to shock if fluids and blood are not replaced quickly.
- *Nerve damage.* This can show up as either numbness or chronic pain. Any numbness—caused when tiny nerves are traumatized—eventually disappears as the nerves heal. But a burning or tearing sensation in the suctioned area may last months.
- *Fat embolism.* When fat is prodded free by the suctioning process, it can slip into the bloodstream and travel to vital organs, causing a potentially fatal blockage. This is extremely rare, though.

71

| COMMON TERM | TECHNICAL TERM | WHAT IS IT? | OPERATION TIME | LIFE OF OPERATION | RECOVERY TIME | PRICE RANGE |
|---|---|---|---|---|---|---|
| Face-lift | Rhytidectomy or Rhytidoplasty | Excess skin is removed from face. Underlying muscles and remaining skin are stretched and tightened. | 3–4 hours | 5–7 years | 2 weeks | $2,500–$5,000 |
| Nose Surgery | Rhinoplasty | Bone and cartilage are reconstructed and excess removed from nose to reshape. | 1–1½ hours | permanent | 1 week | $2,000–$3,000 |
| Eyelid Lift, Eye Surgery | Blepharoplasty | The elimination of fat and excess skin around the eye removes wrinkles, bags, and pouches. | 1½ hours | upper: 10 years; lower: permanent | 1 week | $2,000–$3,000 |
| Eyebrow Lift | Brow Pexy | A section of skin is removed just above the sagging area of the eyebrow, and outer portion of the eyebrow is lifted. | 45 minutes | 10 years | 1 week | $800–$1,200 |
| Ear Surgery | Otoplasty | The cartilage of protruding ears is reshaped, thus repositioning or "pinning back" the ears. | 1½–2 hours | permanent | 1 week | $1,500–$3,000 |
| Forehead Lift | Forehead Lift | Lines and wrinkles are modified through removing excess skin and tightening and stretching remaining skin. Most often performed prior to the need for a full face-lift. | 2 hours | 10 years | 2 weeks | $2,500–$3,500 |
| Chin Surgery, Chin | Mentoplasty | The implantation of a small-grade silicone implant to aug- | 45 minutes | permanent | 1 week | $1,000–$1,500 |

| | | | | | | |
|---|---|---|---|---|---|---|
| Augmentation | | ment receding chin. Often performed with a rhinoplasty to improve profile. | | | | |
| Collagen Implant | Collagen Implant | An injection of the body's natural structural protein, collagen, raises and puffs the skin, smoothing out isolated wrinkles and small scars. | 2 minutes each injection | 3 months–2 years | 2–3 hours | $800–$1,000 first visit $300–$350 each follow-up injection after 6–8 month period. |
| Double-Chin Surgery | Submental Lipectomy | Fat deposits beneath the chin, which result in the "double chin," are removed and the underlying muscles and skin of the upper neck are tightened. | 45 minutes | permanent | 1 week | $800–$1,500 |
| Face Sanding | Dermabrasion | With a wire brush, the face is gently rubbed, removing the outer layer of skin, giving the face a smoother texture. This technique is performed to remove superficial scars and age lines. | 1 hour (full face) | usually permanent | 7–10 days | $1,500–$2,500 |
| Chemical Peel | Chemabrasion | Through a controlled burn with a caustic solution, the outer layer of skin is removed, giving the face a smoother texture. This technique is performed to remove superficial scars and age lines. | 1 hour (full face) | usually permanent | 7–10 days | $1,500–$2,500 |

Courtesy of the American Academy of Facial Plastic and Reconstructive Surgery

One of the beauties of suction lipectomy is that it can be combined with more conventional surgical procedures to achieve an even more pleasing result. Take the tummy tuck, for example. Women with a little looseness of the skin and some slackness in their abdominal muscles can undergo fat suction followed by a new operation called a mini-abdominoplasty. An eight-inch incision is made just above the pubic line and underlying muscles are surgically tightened with sutures up to the navel. Excess skin is then trimmed away. A full abdominoplasty is in order for women with extra fat, very loose skin, and very weak muscles. In this case, a hip-to-hip incision is made just above the pubic area. Skin is freed from the abdominal wall to just below the rib cage, the navel is freed up, and the abdominal muscles are tightened all the way to the ribs. Excess fat is then suctioned and excess skin removed.

## Eyes

Plastic surgeons are now vaporizing the fat inside "baggy eyes" to melt away those unsightly pouches. Under local anesthetic, an electrically heated needle is inserted into the eye bag and the fat cells, which are 90 percent water, simply evaporate! Because there's no actual cutting with a scalpel, the new technique greatly reduces postoperative bleeding and eliminates the risk of blindness, according to its pioneer, Michael Sachs, M.D., of the New York Eye and Ear Infirmary. The cost is $2,000 to $3,000, depending on the size of the bags.

## Nose

An amazing new glue is revolutionizing nose surgery. It's quicker, safer, and the results are far superior to those achieved with conventional techniques. Until now, surgeons have had to resort to a battery of different methods to give noses a more appealing shape. They've implanted fat and silicone and performed bone grafts—all held in place by sutures and steel wires.

That picture has changed now, however, with the introduction of a clear synthetic glue called enbucrilate. Doctors remove tiny pieces of tissue or cartilage from different parts of the patient's own nose—or, occasionally, from the hip or ribs—and sculpt them into the desired shape and size, using this special glue to bond the pieces together. Then a small incision is made in the roof of the nose, via the nostrils, and the implant is carefully inserted. Once it is in place, a little more glue is applied to firmly bind it to existing cartilage, tissue, or bone. The skin fits snugly over this natural implant and the result is an attractive new shape. No external incisions, no sutures, no pieces of steel wire, no silicone, and no fat implants! The glue eventually dissolves and is replaced by natural tissue.

One who finds the results particularly exciting is New York plastic surgeon Thomas Romo, who reports: "Operating time is cut by half, healing is four times as fast as conventional nose jobs, and patients can resume their normal activities within two or three weeks compared with five or six months in the past."[5]

## Face

By far the most common target for plastic surgeons is the face. And our age group is the one most requesting such treatment.

Several procedural advances have improved the results and durability of face-lifts. One technique involves increasing the amount of skin that is actually lifted and tightened. By starting the incision closer to the cheekbone, in front of the ear, and removing more skin, surgeons have been able to make a face-lift last longer. Another improvement is the SMAS (superficial musculo-aponeurotic system) technique. The SMAS is the layer of tissue under the skin that overlies the facial muscles. When the SMAS layer and the skin are lifted and tightened together, the results look better and last longer—because the SMAS is stronger and less elastic than the skin. Such face-lifts can last five years longer than conventional ones.

Surgeons can now work wonders to restore the sharp angle between the chin and the neck. Using techniques similar to the SMAS lift, they can tighten the platysma—a thin, superficial neck muscle at the edge of the jaw—creating a youthful neckline.

Full face-lifts are no longer the norm. Often just upper-face or neck lifts or the removal of loose skin is all that's required. Doing a bit at a time certainly helps financially, too.

## Stretch Marks

Barring accidents, most of us have now put childbearing behind us. Those white or bluish lines on the buttocks, thighs, abdomen, hips, or breasts are also caused by excessive weight gain in adolescence or at any age and also by stretching of the skin during pregnancy.

If you're upset by stretch marks, don't fall prey to bogus promises and false claims. No cream or medication has yet been developed that'll get rid of them. Plastic surgeons have still to come up with a simple and effective technique to eliminate them. A rather drastic method currently being tested is mechanical peeling with dermabrasion.

## Cellulite: No Easy Answer

Controversy still rages in the medical community over the existence of cellulite. While some doctors accept that the orange-peel-like dimpling we're now developing on our thighs and buttocks is no ordinary fat, others maintain it's just that. Fat by any other name is still fat, they say. Whatever it is, we all know it can be unsightly. And that's why a major industry has sprung up to convince us that it can be easily eradicated.

Just look at the advertisements in the back of women's magazines. There's everything from enzymes, creams, hormones, and nutritional supplements to special washcloths. Even beauty salons offer high-priced electrical stimulators, vibrating machines, pressurized suits, herbal wraps, and enzyme injections.

Despite all the hype, there's only one tried and true method to rid yourself of that dimpling: eat less and exercise more. As the excess fat in your body disappears, so will those nasty lumps. Exercises that work the lower body muscles—brisk walking, bicycling, jogging, aerobic dancing—are best, because they not only burn off fat but also help tighten the muscles in our thighs and buttocks.

## Acne

At our age? Ridiculous as it may seem, acne is far from unusual in women our age. However, unlike the adolescent variety, which is generally caused by excessive oiliness, adult acne is associated with seborrheic dermatitis—a dry, dandruff-like condition of the scalp and the creases around the nose and chin.

In the past twenty years there's been an upsurge in adult-onset acne. And the most striking increase is among women who've had a history of going on and off oral contraceptives. The reason: such a pattern of behavior is thought to cause a hormone imbalance in the skin's oil glands, whereby the oil duct thickens, trapping oil and creating pimples and blackheads. When the oil is infected by bacteria, it is transformed into free fatty acids—irritants that cause "explosions" in the clogged oil glands. These explosions are what we commonly call pimples. When the skin's pores become plugged with a combination of oil and dead skin cells, that blockage is known as a blackhead.

A common variety of adult-onset acne is known as acne cosmetica and is triggered by certain skin-care products. Most moisturizers that claim to retard the aging process, for example, are nothing but combinations of oil and water. Not only do they not contain any magical ingredients, but those that contain too much oil can actually be harmful. This type of acne can also be aggravated by the use of oil-base foundations that clog the pores.

Antibiotics are the mainstay of treatment for all acne. They kill pimple-causing bacteria. The best approach is to start treatment with a combination of oral and topical antibiotics for a month or so and then switch to external antibiotics alone. The biggest problem with antibiotic skin creams and lotions is that they are alcohol-based to dry the oily skin of adolescent acne. This can make them irritating to more mature skin. Women our age are usually better off using a new formulation of the antibiotic erythromycin in an ointment base designed for adult skin. Another way of avoiding skin irritation is to use a sulphur cream. Its effectiveness can be enhanced by combining it with salicylic acid.

Other treatments present different problems. Potent cortisone creams quickly clear up much of the inflammation caused by acne, but after a few weeks we tend to become immune to their positive effects. The immunity is soon followed by a rebound to an even more severe case of acne, thus producing a new syndrome known as steroid acne. You're much better off using low-potency steroids, which don't have this side effect.

Probably the most effective treatment for the kind of acne which causes unsightly cysts on the face or back is the retinoid known as accutane. Use of this drug has been linked to birth defects in the offspring of users so it is crucial that users do not become pregnant. Dermatologists use it with great care and with very good effect.

## SKIN SCAMS

I'd be remiss if I were to close this chapter without saying a word or two about skin-care products that simply don't work. While some of them are very effective, many lotions, creams, and treatments—especially those aimed at rejuvenating the skin—are definitely not. And we all need to be on our guard. Remember: if it sounds too good to be true, it probably is. Here's a quick rundown:

*Vitamin-E creams.* To hear some people tell it, Vitamin E is nature's cure-all. Studies have shown that it may help prevent certain detrimental cellular changes in the body that occur with aging. But simply applying Vitamin E to the skin is not only a waste of time; it can actually cause contact dermatitis due to allergies, and outbreaks of acne.

*Hormonal creams.* The assumption is that female hormones firm and smooth the skin and help keep it moist by retaining water. But there's absolutely no sound scientific evidence for this. In fact, emollient creams—costing far less—do a better job.

*Mink oil.* What's so special about mink, unless you're wearing the pelts? Nothing, according to the American Medical Association. *Any* oil applied to the skin will soften it and relieve dryness—and for a lot less money than oil of mink! Remember, no cosmetic preparation—whether it contains mink oil, turtle oil, royal jelly, or any other exotic ingredient—will provide youth and beauty.

*Collagen creams.* While collagen implants work wonders in reducing wrinkles, simply smearing collagen cream on the skin has no effect. The outer layer of skin acts as a barrier that keeps most substances from getting to the deeper skin levels.

Every woman wants to look her best, and now that youth has passed us by, it's important not to panic. We don't have to resort to unproven treatments to preserve the beauty we feel inside. Medical researchers are working to solve some of the many remaining problems in understanding skin conditions and continue to test new products for dermatological care. Keep current with new skin treatments as they are written up in the future and discuss them with your doctor. The very best advice to you is to stay out of the damaging rays of the sun. Be good to your skin!

# 4

# Toward a New Sexuality

More sexual taboos have been put aside in the past twenty-five years than at any other time in history. And I'm glad they have. For too long, sex was something we never spoke about in public—and only rarely in private. The sad result of such repression was that women were kept in the dark about their own sexuality; ignorance of their own bodies brought fear . . . or worse.

Thank God for the sixties! Sex came out of the closet. Women began to be aware of their bodies. We were developing an insatiable appetite for information about our sexuality—a demand that shows no signs of abating. The shackles of repression were being hurled to the wind. Sex was fun! Sex was for everyone! Love-ins were hip. Remember? It was such a release to be able to talk openly about SEX. Birth control was new. We could be spontaneous. If we wanted to make love on the spur of the moment, we could do it without worrying about what would happen nine months down the pike. Great days!

Today we're reaping the benefits of the sexual revolution. Bowing to pressure from women everywhere, the medical profession has not been slow to recognize the need for specialized health care. So, with the sexual revolution has also come a revolution of sorts in the amount of attention being focused on women's health. That's one point for progress. The sexual revolution has also brought problems—which we are only now realizing, years later: an increase in sexually transmitted diseases and consequent greater incidence in infertility. So, a mixed blessing. More about the problems later.

# THE PILL

No other single development has had a more far-reaching impact on the lives of women than the oral contraceptive. Still, it remains controversial. The Pill has been blamed for causing some serious medical problems, from heart attacks to strokes. Every week, it seems, a new study comes out about the Pill. But there is more and more evidence that the oral contraceptive is beneficial to women in more ways than one. So where do we stand?

## Putting the Risks in Perspective

With twenty-five years of experience under our belts, we now have a much better handle on the impact oral contraceptives have upon our bodies. That's important, because you and I are now at the age when we're going to develop those health problems that the Pill has been blamed for in the past. And some of us have been taking it for more than half our lives.

According to a recent nationwide poll, many American women think that oral contraceptives are more hazardous than having a baby! But that's far from the truth. A new study, concerned with illness caused by the Pill in a group of 35,000 women, found that there were some instances of blood clots in the legs, but no woman died from the side effects of the Pill, nor was it related to strokes or heart attacks. These results contrasted

81

dramatically with those of earlier studies in which it was demonstrated that there were substantial risks associated with taking the Pill.

Why the difference? The Pill has changed. Twenty-five years ago, it contained amounts of estrogen that, by today's standards, were massive. The pill we've been taking for the past fifteen years has much less of this hormone. And the less synthetic estrogen we can get away with without risking pregnancy, the better, it seems. Today the risk of serious complications is very slim.

To get back to that nationwide poll I mentioned, how *do* the risks of taking the Pill compare with those of having a baby? Well, despite modern medicine, childbirth is still potentially dangerous. For a woman between the ages of twenty and twenty-five, it's at least twice as hazardous as taking birth-control pills. High blood pressure, hemorrhage, and infection are very definite risks in pregnancy. In women our age, the odds get closer, but they're still in the Pill's favor.

Of course, some women do have problems with the Pill. These include spotting, mood changes, and a slightly increased risk of developing gallstones. But the most serious Pill-related problems occur in women who smoke—and smoking should take most of the blame. Women who smoke are more likely to develop blood clots, whether they take the Pill or not. There is, however, a link between blood clots and the use of birth-control pills by women of our age, whether we smoke or not. Smoking just increases that risk.

The synthetic estrogen in oral contraceptives can also aggravate existing conditions. If you fall into any of the following categories, you should consider a different method of contraception:

- A history of clotting problems—such as phlebitis, stroke, or pulmonary embolism—heart attack, or angina
- Liver disease, such as hepatitis or cirrhosis

- Cancer of the breast or uterus
- Unexplained vaginal bleeding

If you suspect you're pregnant, you should also give up the Pill. In addition, temporarily stop taking oral contraceptives if you have an abdominal operation or must stay in bed because of an injury such as a leg fracture. These factors can predispose you to blood clots. Other conditions do not pose absolute restrictions on using the Pill, but you should discuss them with your doctor. These include diabetes, high blood pressure, migraines, infrequent menstrual periods, and a family history of early heart attacks or uterine or breast cancer.

## Seeing the Bonus Advantages

Besides being 99.26 percent effective in preventing conception, oral contraception has some major health benefits. In fact, it significantly reduces the incidence of no less than seven serious diseases, preventing an estimated fifty thousand hospitalizations a year in the United States.

*Benign breast disease.* The incidence of benign breast disease such as cystic mastitis is reduced 50 to 75 percent by oral contraceptive use.

*Ovarian cysts.* Because the Pill suppresses ovarian function, its use markedly reduces the incidence of certain types of ovarian cysts that may require surgery.

*Pelvic inflammatory disease (PID).* Women using oral contraceptives are one third as likely to develop this widespread infection as those who do not. The Center for Disease Control reckons that the Pill prevents thousands of cases of PID each year. This type of disease, commonly sparked by chlamydia and gonorrhea, is a major cause of sterility.

*Endometrial and ovarian cancer.* Pill users appear to slash their risk of getting these reproductive-tract cancers by more than half. And the protection seems to persist for at least ten years after the Pill is stopped.

83

*Iron-deficiency anemia.* Pill users suffer approximately 45 percent less iron-deficiency anemia, partly due to less blood lost during menstruation.

*Rheumatoid arthritis.* Studies indicate that current users of the Pill are only half as likely to develop rheumatoid arthritis as are nonusers.

In general, then, it is clear that women who have been on the Pill for years have had real benefits to their health as they are very much aware. Because the Pill has been diligently studied for twenty-five years (but not thirty-five!) these statistics I have given you are reassuring. However, there is evidence that risk for heart attack does increase in women over forty on the Pill and significantly for over-forty smokers. For how long can you continue to take it safely? Until you are forty-five? Fifty? We don't know. I advise women of forty and over to review very carefully their other risk factors (see Chapter 7) and to see what their cholesterol and triglyceride levels are: many elect to have a tubal ligation done or change to another birth control method in view of the present state of our knowledge. Keep yourself informed about new developments in the media concerning this topic and keep in touch with your doctor.[1]

## The Abortion Pill Is Here!

By 1990, the first abortion pill is expected to be available in the United States. It's already being used in Europe, having recently received the blessing of the French government. But, as abortion has always been a thorny issue in America, it will likely face a good deal of stiff opposition here before we're allowed to put it to use.

Developed in France, the drug has safely and easily induced abortions in 85 percent of women who take it within ten days of missing a menstrual period. If the U.S. Food and Drug Administration gives the nod, this pill will revolutionize abortion in this country—taking it out of the abortion clinic and placing it firmly in the hands of a woman and her own doctor, which, in my opinion, is where it belongs.

There are major differences between the abortion pill, known as RU486, and contraceptives or morning-after pills. With the contraceptive pill, the egg produced in the ovaries each month is not released, so it can't be fertilized. The morning-after pill prevents a fertilized egg from implanting and growing on the wall of the uterus. But the new pill solves the problem of fertilized eggs that have actually implanted in the womb. It blocks release of progesterone, which is vital for the development of the embryo. Without progesterone, the fertilized egg decays and is passed from the body through menstrual bleeding—as in a miscarriage. This usually occurs within two weeks of taking the new drug. Side effects are minimal—usually cramps and a heavy menstrual flow.

All one hundred women in the French study were scheduled for surgical abortion. Having taken this pill, eighty-five did not need to undergo surgery. So it certainly appears to be a safe and effective alternative.

Clearly, RU486 has major implications for women all over the world. Abortion, as we know it today, will more or less disappear in the near future. That's not just wishful thinking; it's a distinct probability now.

Decision making will be much easier for a woman because her own doctor will be able to prescribe the drug and she will not have to face the trauma of entering the often cold, impersonal atmosphere of the abortion clinic.

## STERILIZATION

Now that we're in our forties, many of us are reassessing our method of birth control. Although there's a definite swing toward later pregnancy, millions of women are deciding that forty is a good time to opt for sterilization: no pills, no IUDs, no condoms.

Sterilization is now the leading form of birth control in the world and the choice of almost twelve million Americans. Every year, half a million men and 750,000 women elect this permanent form of contraception. It does, after all, have many advantages over other methods: it's the most reliable, the risk of death or complications is extremely low, and once you've had it done, you need never worry about contraception again. The only disadvantages are its irreversibility and the initial cost, which ranges from $100 to $2,000.

Voluntary sterilization means deciding to give up forever the capacity to reproduce, regardless of events such as divorce and remarriage, or the death of your children or spouse. You must be certain that no matter what happens in your life, you never want to have another child. If there's the slightest doubt, don't go through with it, because there are no guarantees that it can be successfully reversed—although progress is definitely being made in that direction.

Sterilization in men is far easier to perform, less expensive, and involves a much lower risk of surgical complications than does female sterilization. The vasectomy costs about $400, is performed under local anesthetic in a doctor's office, and usually takes only twenty minutes. Reversal in men is very much more successful than in women. Some urologists say that male fertility returns in 90 percent of cases after reversal surgery.

For women, the most popular sterilization technique is laparoscopy—often called "belly-button" or "Band-Aid" surgery because of the tiny incision that's made just inside the navel and covered later by a small dressing. The twenty-minute procedure is quicker and less expensive than the more conventional tubal-ligation operation, which can cost as much as $2,000.

Once the incision is made, carbon-dioxide gas is pumped in to distend the abdomen, giving the physician more room to work without risk of damage to other organs. Through the same tiny slit, a long, hollow, pencil-thin tube is inserted. It has a light source at its tip and magnifying mirrors that allow the physician to see the internal organs clearly. He can then

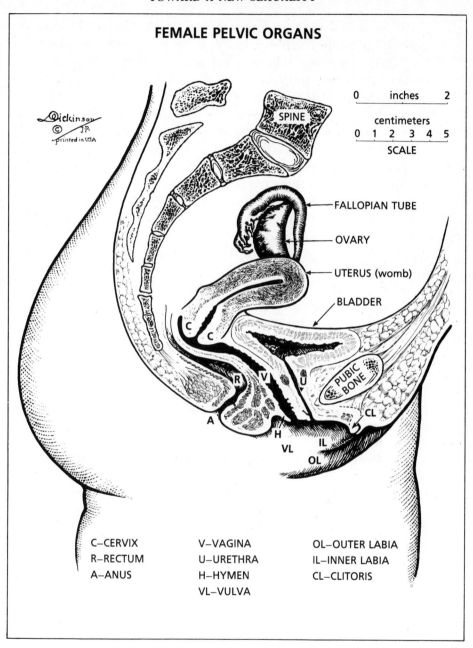

## FEMALE PELVIC ORGANS

C–CERVIX      V–VAGINA      OL–OUTER LABIA
R–RECTUM    U–URETHRA    IL–INNER LABIA
A–ANUS       H–HYMEN      CL–CLITORIS
              VL–VULVA

87

insert special surgical instruments through the tube or through a second, equally small incision just above the pubic hairline. For sterilization, the fallopian tubes are either cauterized or pulled into a tiny loop and sealed with a clip or ring fitted around the neck of the loop. Sealing each fallopian tube permanently prevents any meeting between sperm and egg, so conception cannot occur. After the tubes are closed off, the instruments are removed and the incisions closed.

Complications are rare, and a two- to four-hour rest in a hospital or a clinic afterward is usually all that's required. Most women can return to work in two to five days. Cost of the operation varies from around $450 to $1,000.

The chance of a successful reversal varies according to the type of procedure performed. Tubes that are cauterized suffer more damage than those sealed with a clip and are therefore far more difficult to reopen; thus, doctors often recommend the latter method, especially for women who are likely to seek a reversal—those who are single or who are unsure that their marriage will last.

Today, the pregnancy rate after reversal is about 65 percent for the ring method. But this high degree of success is being achieved only by top surgeons operating on carefully selected patients. For women whose tubes are cauterized, the success rate drops dramatically. Cost of a reversal operation is between $5,000 and $6,000.

It's encouraging to know that fewer than 10 percent of sterilized women eventually regret their decision and seek a reversal. Clearly, the overwhelming majority opt for this ultimate form of birth control only after thoughtful consideration and adequate education about all the pros and cons. Many women report that it injects a tremendous sense of freedom into their lives and gives them much more satisfying sex because they no longer have fears of an unwanted pregnancy.

# SEX AFTER FORTY

Reflecting on our own sexuality, many of us will recall with amusement the perception we had as youngsters about our parents' sex lives. Remember thinking that no one over forty could possibly have a sex life?

While aging does bring about certain physical changes, sexual fulfillment is possible at any age, particularly with today's advances in medicine, greater emphasis on fitness and health, and increased self-awareness.

In women, estrogen loss at menopause causes dryness of the vagina which can be treated successfully with topical hormone creams. Vaginal muscle tone may also relax with age but can be restored by doing Kegel exercises—tightening and then relaxing vaginal muscles twenty to thirty times a day (see page 95).

Eating nutritionally well and sticking to a program of exercise are important, too, for good sex after forty. It stands to reason that if you feel good about your body, you'll enjoy sex more—whether you're eighteen or eighty-one.

Years ago, decreased libido or sex drive was known to be a problem for middle-aged men stressed by the business world and the financial responsibilities of a family entirely dependent on them. Times have changed, and women now experience these same career stresses and resultant loss of interest in sex which is puzzling to them. Whether a single parent or a working mother, it is easier for us to understand a boyfriend or husband being "too tired" after a hard day at work because we share this experience. This sharing should be able to bring a couple closer together sexually, if they set time apart for themselves in their busy lives.

## Rx for the Sexual Blahs

Michele, forty-two, came to see me one day. She'd just returned to work as an office manager after spending the past fifteen years at home raising her children. "I find the work and responsibility really satisfying," she said, "but when I get home at night, I'm so tired I just have no interest in sex. Bob is starting to complain and I'm really worried."

Loss of sexual desire is common today in women who are "doing it all," juggling a rising career with the demands of a partner and adolescent children, extended family and social responsibilities. Sexual desire is a human appetite or drive expressed as interest in sexual experience. It is produced by the physical activation of an identified anatomical neural system in the brain: it is separate from the arousal, excitement and orgasmic phases of sexual response, which involve the genital organs and work from a different circuit in the brain.

The sexual drive is balanced between activation and inhibition. Activation by signals received by the brain center to stimulate desire is easier to understand than inhibition. The full chemical and neurological mechanisms are not yet completely understood, but it is known that inhibition can be caused by physiological factors such as hormonal changes, illness, drugs (including alcohol), stress, depression and pain, and by psychological factors such as anger, hostility to the partner, being turned off by the appearance or behavior of the partner, deep-seated unconscious feelings and conflicts, anxiety and fear— fear of failing in performance, fear of intimacy, fear of danger.[2] A simple example is thinking you hear a burglar downstairs. The ear flashes a signal to the brain which sends the message on to the neural center of initiation of sexual desire. "Cool it!" the message reads—"now is not the time." This is a healthy and appropriate protective mechanism. It can, for example, remind you that the good-looking man on your right is married to the woman on your left.

But when anxiety suppresses libido all or most of the time or at the wrong times then it becomes a problem. It's important to try to pinpoint the causes of anxiety or stress.

- Have you been experiencing fears about your health or appearance? A painful disease, such as arthritis, or concern about aging, changes in your looks, or weight gain may be at the root of the problem.

- Have you been quarreling with the kids? Sexual desire is often stifled by mother/daughter conflicts.
- Have you had a breakdown of communication with your partner? A surefire impediment to sexual desire is a lack of conversation or understanding. Learning to talk to each other again is vitally important.
- Have you or your partner been diagnosed as having a heart condition or high blood pressure? Many people are frightened into abandoning sex. Yet, studies show that people rarely die during intercourse and that, indeed, the stress caused by restricting sex can be worse than the risks posed by continuing to enjoy it.
- Are you having to take on new responsibilities?

In some cases, inhibition of desire is a more difficult issue involving deep-seated fears and anxieties. Sexual dysfunction is often treated today by a new technique called psychosexual therapy. The couple is assigned to do structured sexual tasks at home; then, together they see the therapist once a week in the office. The sexual exercises are discussed in detail during the therapy sessions, with special attention focused on the emotional feelings, as well as physical reactions, evoked in each partner by these experiences. Anxieties, conflicts, and especially resistances brought out during these discussions are then fully explored.

Through counseling, Michele found that the extra energy required for her new job drained her of sexual energy. So she and her husband worked out a new set of expectations and priorities: by setting aside time for themselves, the problem cleared up.

Analysis and treatment of sexual dysfunction are still in their infancy. What we've discovered so far represents probably less than a third of the variants in understanding loss of sexual desire. But doors are now being opened. Loss of desire should no longer be an affliction that leaves the sufferer feeling isolated and hopeless. It *can* be treated.

## Painful Intercourse

"Why does it hurt when I have sex?" Helen asked when she came to see me. "My husband and I have always had a good sex life, but now I'm losing interest because intercourse hurts so much. Please help: it's affecting our marriage."

After vaginal discharge, painful intercourse is the sexual problem most often reported by women today. And it can almost always be easily cured—with drugs or surgery, depending on the cause.

When women in their early to mid-forties have painful sex, it's usually from an infection or the results of pregnancy or delivery:

- Vulvitis, vaginitis, and cervicitis are common inflammations seen in women. The resulting redness and soreness of the outer genital area or vagina and frequent irritating discharge are cleared up by using appropriate antibiotics.
- Pelvic inflammatory disease (PID) is caused by various infections of the fallopian tubes and ovaries. Symptoms include abdominal tenderness, fever, vaginal discharge, loss of appetite. Aggressive antibiotic therapy is essential; surgery may be necessary.
- Endometriosis, a painful condition of the pelvis that often prevents pregnancy, is occasionally seen in older women who've delayed childbearing. It's a disease that usually responds to hormonal therapy, surgery, or, more recently, laser therapy.
- Scars from pelvic surgery or a difficult forceps delivery may occasionally make coitus uncomfortable.

In menopausal women, sexual discomfort is often the result of a dry vagina, caused by decreased hormone levels. Many women have found that using a simple lubricant during intercourse—K-Y Jelly—brings safe relief. During orgasm, menopausal women experience fewer pelvic spasms and return more quickly to a relaxed state than do younger women. Occasionally, however, the genital muscular contractions that occur during orgasm can be prolonged and cause cramps.

Also, as the vaginal walls are less capable of stretching than before, intercourse may cause small, painful tears. Additionally, with the thinning of these walls, the urethra—the tube that carries urine from the bladder—may be irritated by the thrusting of the penis. This often results in a burning sensation during urination, more frequent urination for two or three days after intercourse, and, occasionally, cramps in the lower abdomen or bloating. Using an estrogen cream in the vagina once a week can reverse the dryness and thinness of the walls (see Chapter 5). Estrogen pills may help, too.

## No Play: You Pay

Regular sex can compensate for the physiological changes in the vagina. Researchers at the Rutgers Medical School[3] found that women in their forties and fifties who are sexually active suffer less vaginal deterioration than those who enjoy sex infrequently. They recommend we have intercourse at least three times a month—to tone up our vaginas!

## Pelvic-Support Problems

Childbirth—and the trauma it causes to tissues—leaves women in their thirties and forties particularly vulnerable to pelvic-support problems that interfere with enjoyable sex. A "dropped," or prolapsed, uterus or a sagging bladder or urethra commonly result from relaxation of the muscular and ligamentous support. Tissue fibers become so stretched and thin that they separate and tear. Already weakened tissue may be strained further by obesity. And age-related estrogen depletion compounds the problem, so that a menopausal woman with a slightly dropped uterus may have a very serious prolapse by age sixty-five.

There are four common types of pelvic-relaxation problems:

*Cystocele* is a prolapse of the bladder into the vaginal canal. A lump or bulge commonly appears just inside the vaginal opening. It's particularly noticeable when the woman stands, because the weight of urine forces the bladder to protrude even further. Over time, urinary difficulties develop. In severe cases, the bladder sags below the urethral outlet, so urine must be forced uphill before being expelled. Consequently, the bladder does not empty completely and becomes a breeding ground for infection. Surgically repairing the vaginal wall is the treatment of choice.

*Uterine prolapse* occurs when the uterus descends into the vaginal canal. With minimal descent, there may be no symptoms. More pronounced prolapse is often first detected by a sexual partner who finds deep penile penetration blocked. The condition can worsen until the entire uterus actually protrudes outside the vagina. Since a dropped uterus will pull on the bladder and urethra, urinary difficulties occur, as do bladder infections caused by retained urine.

A hysterectomy is usually recommended when the condition is causing distress. At the same time, any sagging of the vaginal walls, urethra, and bladder can be corrected. In young women who may want more children, the operation can be delayed.

*Rectocele* is a protrusion of the rectal wall into the vaginal canal. It causes little discomfort, although there may be difficulty in fully emptying the rectum. Women with this condition often find relief by inserting a finger into the vagina and pressing the back wall to facilitate evacuation. Surgery corrects the problem and restores function to normal.

*Urethrocele* is a condition in which the urethra, instead of being tucked against the pubic bone, sags downward, causing stress incontinence—the involuntary expulsion of urine when laughing or sneezing. Depending on the severity of the problem, the urethra can be resuspended in its normal position surgically or through special muscle exercises.

## Sexercises

When you're physically fit, you can do everything better—including making love. There's no substitute for overall body conditioning and regular exercise. But did you know there's a set of special exercises that may help heighten sexual feeling? Called Kegel exercises, they are directed at strengthening the pelvic muscles by rhythmically contracting and relaxing them.

The first set of exercises is to contract the pelvic muscles tightly for five seconds, then relax for five. Repeat the pattern at least ten times. Next, contract and relax the muscles as rapidly as you can for a count of five. Rest, then repeat the exercise. This can easily be done in bed before dropping off to sleep, while driving the car, or even while sitting at the movies.

Second, try to stop the flow of urination by squeezing the muscles of the pelvic floor as tightly as possible. Once you are able to stop the flow, practice starting and stopping it until it becomes easy to do. This may be difficult or even impossible at first, but, believe me, it can be achieved with practice. Your patience will be rewarded with better bladder control.

Try to do these exercises as often as possible. For maximum sexual enhancement, you need to be doing them up to fifty times a day for two to three weeks and then at least once a week thereafter. By strengthening the muscles that contract during orgasm, you'll be giving yourself a sexual tune-up and adding to the pleasure experienced by both you and your partner.

# PREGNANCY AT OUR AGE

In the past fifteen years, planned pregnancies among women in their thirties and forties have tripled. They now account for 10 percent of the total number. And the figure's rising all the time. Of course, pregnancy at our age has some distinct advantages: we have more money than we did twenty years ago, our careers and life-styles are set, and we just feel more comfortable about life. Our heads are, well, more together now. So why not start a family?

As we all know, there are increased risks in having a baby at our age. But, that said, major technological advances are giving physicians a battery of new devices and new tests that can often spot a developing problem in time for it to be treated. Just one mind-blowing example: not too long ago, a team of California surgeons removed a twenty-three-week-old fetus from his mother's womb, successfully operated to correct a blocked urinary tract, and then returned the unborn baby to the uterus and sewed it back up. Nine weeks later, Baby Mitchell was born alive and well!

## Getting Pregnant

Peak fertility age for a woman is twenty-four. And as the years pass by, the chances of becoming pregnant diminish. Women under thirty who want to conceive have a 90 percent chance of becoming pregnant within a year, while those over thirty-five usually have to try a little longer.

Sometimes it's simply a matter of timing intercourse to coincide precisely with ovulation. A number of portable devices are on the market now to help. One of them, the Cue Monitor, can accurately predict ovulation four to six days before actual release of the egg. So you have plenty of time to get in the right frame of mind! The device measures subtle changes in the electrical signals that pass between the brain and the ovaries. It takes only ten seconds to get a reading from the monitor—a lot less than with some others that are available. These types of monitors are now being made available to physicians, who can rent them out to patients with infertility problems.

If you're having difficulty getting pregnant, it may not be a gynecological problem, of course. After all, infertility is not just a problem of women alone. Help is at hand. Doctors have now found a way of strengthening sperm so it has the "muscle" to make that long swim to fertilize the egg. It's not the quantity of sperm a man ejaculates but the quality that counts. At the Fertility Institute of Western Massachusetts, they're giving sperm a special high-protein meal, then selecting those that are the strongest swimmers for implantation into the woman's uterus. Sounds comical, but it's worked in 35 percent of cases!

## In Search of Fertility

Reproductive medicine is making tremendous strides in helping women of all ages become pregnant. But what should you expect when you visit a specialist in infertility?

A good infertility workup begins with a thorough physical examination and blood and hormone tests. You'll be asked to record your morning body temperature, which changes as your ovaries prepare to release an egg each month.

To determine if your fallopian tubes are open and normal, a tubal insufflation test is performed, whereby carbon dioxide is introduced into the uterus and the tubes. With a stethoscope, the physician will listen for gas escaping into the abdomen. To pinpoint blockages, special X rays are taken as dye is injected into the uterus and fallopian tubes (hysterosalpingogram). Both procedures are usually done between the seventh and the tenth day of a woman's twenty-eight-day menstrual cycle.

A postcoital test is another possibility. It's performed around the thirteenth day of the cycle. Mucus taken from the cervix six to fourteen hours after intercourse is examined for the presence of moving, living sperm. A negative result may indicate that the mucus is too thick, the sperm is of poor quality, or there are chemical incompatibilities.

Around the twentieth day of the cycle, after ovulation has presumably occurred, an endometrial biopsy can be performed. A tiny sample of the lining of the uterus is obtained and examined to see if the uterus's preparation for pregnancy is in sync with ovulation.

When these tests don't reveal any abnormalities, more advanced testing is needed. Minor surgical procedures such as laparoscopy and culdoscopy allow a physician to look directly at a woman's internal organs for evidence of disease causing infertility.

Infertility can be a difficult puzzle to solve; therefore, it's important for couples to remember that fertility is cyclic—it varies each month and is not constant. The same test may have to be conducted several times before a specific problem can be ruled out.

Intermittent or nonexistent ovulation is one of the most common causes of infertility. Clearly, if no egg is produced, there can be no baby. It is possible to have normal menstrual cycles without ovulating. The easiest way to tell if you're ovulating is to take your temperature every morning. A small dip followed by a larger rise is evidence that ovulation has occurred.

Although slightly uncomfortable, the best ovulation detection technique is the biopsy of the uterine lining I have just described. Performed several days after ovulation, the endometrial response to progesterone is unmistakable under the microscope.

A number of steps can be taken to help a woman who's not ovulating. Sometimes the thyroid gland fails to produce sufficient thyroid hormone. A blood test can detect this deficiency, and hormone-replacement therapy may prove successful. Anovulation associated with an overproduction of the pituitary hormone prolactin has been treated successfully with a drug called bromocriptine or Parlodel—ovulating cycles resulted in about 75 percent of women who were treated with this drug.

Women who are not ovulating can often be helped by a drug called clomiphene citrate. It's a remarkable medicine: 70 percent of women who take it ovulate and 40 percent conceive. The drug is taken for five days, starting three to five days after a period begins. The dosage varies from woman to woman: some require one tablet a day, others four or more. At higher doses side effects such as hot flashes, vascular headaches, or visual changes can occur.

Another technique to stimulate the ovary is the injection of the pituitary hormones, LH and FSH. These are sold under the trade name Pergonal. This drug caused multiple pregnancies in 20 percent of women treated for induction of ovulation. While most of these were twins, the risks to both mother and infants of triplets, quadruplets, and other multiple pregnancies must be carefully considered.

Careful monitoring of the patient is therefore necessary to prevent, if possible, overstimulation of the ovaries and the release of more than one egg, leading to a multiple pregnancy.

## Reducing Pregnancy Risks

The last twenty-five years have seen a dramatic change in maternal and child health statistics in America: maternal deaths have plummeted to less than 280 from 1,500 annually and infant mortality has dropped from 256 to below 11 per 1,000 live births in the same time frame. The maternity statistics include women of all ages in all of the United States. So the chances of dying in childbirth are really negligible at any age, especially if women do not have a serious underlying condition such as heart disease, diabetes, or asthma. Women over forty may have more complications of pregnancy as it may, for example, bring on a temporary state of diabetes or be a strain on those with severe varicose veins.

But I don't think these concerns should dissuade you from

starting a family at your age or increasing the size of your present one, given the sophisticated obstetrical care available to you. You would automatically be considered high-risk and be given more tests and check-ups than younger women. Which is excellent. If you decide to go ahead with a pregnancy and you are in your forties, there are some things you need to check out first.

Start by taking a look at your health in general. If your weight and blood pressure are normal, you're already ahead of the game. If you've never smoked, don't start now. If you do smoke, you absolutely must stop during pregnancy, for the sake of your unborn baby.

Examine your family history to see if anyone has had diabetes that began late in life. If there is such a history, your doctor will probably recommend a sugar-tolerance test before you become pregnant or when you're in the early stages of pregnancy.

One major risk of pregnancy after forty is that of birth defects caused by damaged chromosomes—the cell structures containing the genes, which determine our inherited characteristics. It is important to remember that we were born with all the eggs we'll ever have. As we age, so do the egg cells. And the longer they hang around waiting for their turn to be released from the ovaries, the greater the chance of damage to the chromosomes.

The most common defect of this type is Down syndrome (also known as mongolism). A woman who becomes pregnant at forty-five may have as high as one chance in forty-six of having an affected baby. I like to think of this as there being forty-five healthy babies for every one born with a problem. But it is something you should consider very carefully before deciding to have a baby at such an age. Fortunately, other defects are rare. And there's no increased risk at our age of giving birth to a child with one of the many inherited disorders of biochemical metabolism, such as phenylketonuria (PKU), which causes severe mental retardation.

Several tests are now available for women who want a prenatal diagnosis to check for disease and genetic defects. In addition, medical advances such as fetal monitoring have made delivery safer. So it's only a very small percentage of women over forty for whom pregnancy is really dangerous. And with special prenatal care and careful monitoring, the chances are excellent that things will turn out well.

First pregnancies later in life do not necessarily result in longer hours of labor. Nor do they inevitably lead to a Caesarean section. Older mothers can, however, expect a higher rate of miscarriage. It may also take them longer to conceive—ten to twelve months, on average, for a woman over forty, compared with four months for a woman in her twenties.

The incidence of identical twins also goes up with age, as does the chance of having a girl rather than a boy.

Despite the risks, pregnancy is often one of the most rewarding experiences for a woman over forty. Emotionally and financially, we're far better prepared to bring a new life into the world than when we were in our twenties.

## Fetal Monitoring

Fetal monitor machines are making the actual birth of a baby much safer for all women. They record the heart rate of the fetus during labor, as well as measure contractions of the mother's uterus. Together, these show how the baby is responding to the contractions, making your doctor aware of any problems and giving him or her the opportunity to correct them, if possible. This type of monitoring is now used with more than half of the more than three million births that occur in the United States each year. And because at our age we're at a higher than normal risk, it's a probability that our labor will be monitored in this way.

## Diabetes in Pregnancy

Until just a few years ago, being diabetic and pregnant was considered extremely dangerous because of the risk of miscarriage, stillbirth, or birth defects. But the picture's changing.

It is now known that keeping the blood sugars in the normal or physiological range will prevent the complications of high blood sugar in the fetus and reduce the perinatal mortality to that of nondiabetic women. Hyperglycemia in the unborn child leads to excessive fetal growth which increases the risk of stillbirth, birth trauma, Caesarean section, asphyxia, and respiratory distress syndrome in the newborn.

A woman with type I juvenile-onset diabetes must be sure to have the disease under strict control prior to conception and adhere rigorously to her planned regimen of insulin injections, diet, and exercise. Women with type II or noninsulin dependent diabetes, which normally begins at the age of 45–54 and is accelerated by pregnancy, need to pay scrupulous attention to their diet and may need insulin during the pregnancy to maintain normal blood sugars. Pregnancy causes temporary diabetes in 8 percent of women. Risk factors for developing gestational diabetes include a family history of diabetes and/or a history of unexplained miscarriages or stillbirths. If you have had excessive weight gain in pregnancy or a previous delivery resulting in a nine pound-plus birth weight infant, then you are at risk for developing diabetes in pregnancy and should be tested with blood sugar and glucose-tolerance tests.

Once pregnant, a diabetic, as has been noted, needs to have special care in pregnancy. This means close supervision by a diabetes specialist and perinatologist who specializes in high-risk pregnancies. You will need to see your obstetrician more often and be tested more frequently than other women. If the blood sugar level rises too high you may need insulin injections to control the levels for the duration of the pregnancy. If the disease is severe you may be admitted to the hospital for the

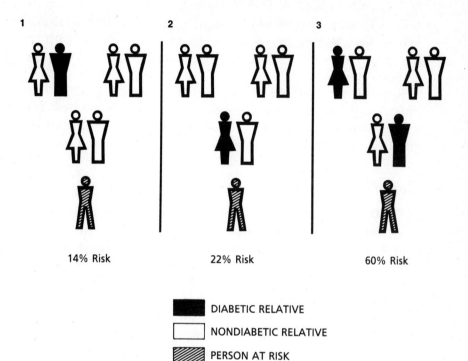

1                    2                    3

14% Risk          22% Risk          60% Risk

■ DIABETIC RELATIVE
☐ NONDIABETIC RELATIVE
▨ PERSON AT RISK

1. If only one of your grandparents had diabetes, you have a 14 percent chance of getting it.
2. If one of your parents (but no other relative) had diabetes, you have a 22 percent chance of getting it.
3. If one of your parents *and* one of your grandparents (or an aunt or uncle) had diabetes, your chances of getting it rise to 60 percent. *The Upjohn Company*

## YOUR RISK OF DEVELOPING DIABETES

last days or weeks of your pregnancy so that the diabetes may be controlled precisely and the baby's condition closely monitored. Failure to keep blood sugar under control may cause ketoacidosis, a condition which may result in sudden death of the fetus. It's clear, isn't it, that gestational diabetes must be taken very seriously.

Remember: controlling diet and sugar levels is of critical importance before and during pregnancy. While medical advances make it possible for you to give birth safely, your health and that of your baby requires your complete cooperation.

## Genetic Counseling

Two to 3 percent of all babies inherit a major physical or mental defect. And the brunt of that risk is borne by women who delay pregnancy into their thirties and forties. Until recently, parents could only worry and wait to see if their child would be normal. Today, however, in many cases doctors may rely on a simple blood test to determine a couple's statistical chances of having a child with a genetic disorder—so they know the risks before the pregnancy starts.

Genetic counseling is recommended for all women in our age group, for couples who have already had a child with a birth defect, or for prospective parents one or both of whom has a family history of a genetic disorder. It is also suggested for workers who have been exposed to radiation or toxic chemicals, people whose medical or psychiatric condition is thought to have a genetic component, and women with a history of miscarriage.

Great progress has been made in the field of genetics in recent years. We can now detect every one of the known chromosomal abnormalities before the baby is born, and we can identify carriers of close to sixty diseases before a baby is conceived. As the number of detectable diseases continues to grow, specialists are beginning to treat many of these disorders in the womb, attempting to provide a cure before birth.

Just as a baby inherits the color of its eyes and hair from its parents, certain types of birth defects are also passed on through the genes and chromosomes. Genetic disorders can be divided into three main categories: those caused by abnormalities in the genes; those caused by too few or too many chromosomes; and those involving a combination of genetic and environmental factors (such as cigarette smoke or alcohol).

The most advanced techniques in the field are those that detect fetal abnormalities in the womb. Of these techniques, the two most widely known are ultrasound and amniocentesis. But other, more sophisticated tests are currently being studied at many major hospitals.

*Ultrasound* uses sound waves to create a picture of the fetus. This technique is used to examine the size and sex of the fetus and to look for any defects. The placenta, its size and position, is also studied. The sound waves can't be heard, because they're beyond our hearing range. But they're able to pass through the skin and are reflected off surfaces of the fetus, producing a pattern of dots and spaces that can be pictured on a video screen.

*Amniocentesis* is most valuable for detecting chromosome abnormalities, such as those responsible for Tay-Sachs disease, sickle-cell anemia, and Down syndrome. The test involves, simply, taking a sample from the fluid-filled amniotic sac—the bag of waters—that surrounds the fetus. The risk of miscarriage or other serious problems developing from amniocentesis is very small—less than 1 percent. Perhaps the most exciting new use for amniocentesis is intrauterine blood transfusion for a fetus severely affected by Rh blood disease (erythroblastosis). A baby too premature to survive delivery—and likely to die in the uterus—can be given a life-saving blood transfusion while still inside the mother's womb.

New tests are cutting down on that wait-and-worry time. There are two that are capturing a lot of attention: CVS (chorionic villus sampling) and AFP (alpha-fetoprotein). CVS involves analyzing a small amount of tissue from the placenta, which attaches the fetus to the wall of the uterus. The placenta contains the same cells as the fetus. You have an answer within twenty-four hours on whether or not the fetus is normal. The technique is painless, requires no anesthetic, and can be performed in a doctor's office in less than thirty minutes. The AFP test is even more important. A simple analysis of the mother's blood is all it takes. And it's tipping doctors off to major nervous-system deformities in the unborn baby. Already, California requires that the AFP test be made available to all expectant mothers, and, at present, about one-third of all pregnancies in New England are also being screened in this way.

The test—performed about the sixteenth week of pregnancy—is not surefire yet. But an abnormal result suggests that more elaborate tests, such as ultrasound or amniocentesis, should be considered.

AFP is a protein present in the body of the growing fetus. If there's a defect in the baby's body wall, large amounts of the protein can escape and enter the mother's blood. The test detects any abnormally high levels, indicating that something may be seriously wrong with the baby. The main target is the early detection of neural tube defects in the spine, although the test may also suggest other structural abnormalities. High AFP in the mother's blood can, for instance, indicate an abnormal opening in the abdominal wall which leaves the internal organs exposed. Screening for maternal AFP reportedly detects 90 percent of *anencephaly* (open lesion of the skull) and 60 percent of *spina bifida* (open lesion along the backbone) cases.

A definitive diagnosis of a major birth defect at this stage gives parents the option of terminating the pregnancy. However, if they decide against abortion, doctors will still be better prepared to deal with the defect when the baby is born. AFP testing is rapidly becoming a part of routine prenatal care. The American College of Obstetricians and Gynecologists endorses the test but emphasizes that it should be used only as a part of a comprehensive program that would include patient education.

## Ectopic Pregnancy

Another major concern for those of us older women wishing to have a baby in the near future is the possibility of the fetus developing outside the uterus. Called ectopic, or extrauterine, pregnancy, it's a problem that's increasing because of delayed pregnancies and the epidemic of pelvic infections caused most frequently by chlamydia and gonorrhea which infect and cause swelling and then scarring and obstruction of the tubes. Use of an IUD—intrauterine device—for birth control has also resulted in infection of the uterus and tubes with resultant adhesions and scarring. Since 1970 the number of ectopic pregnancies has quadrupled. Not only that; it's the leading cause of maternal death in the first trimester, and in black women, the leading cause of maternal death—period.

In normal pregnancy, the egg is fertilized by the sperm inside the fallopian tube and then travels to the uterus, where it attaches to the inside wall and begins to grow. In an ectopic pregnancy, the egg remains in the fallopian tube. Because only the uterus is equipped with a proper food supply to nourish the fetus and with an expandable wall that allows the fetus to grow, most ectopic pregnancies either abort or rupture within six weeks. There are extremely rare cases, however, in which the pregnancy goes to term and an infant is delivered by Caesarean section. But the incidence of birth defects in such infants is considerably higher than the norm.

In most ectopic pregnancies, the fallopian tubes are obstructed in such a way that the fertilized egg can't reach the uterus. These obstructions are often the result of pelvic disease, endometriosis (when the uterine lining grows outside the uterus), scar tissue from previous pelvic surgery, fibroid tumors pressing against the tubes, or a congenital deformity.

The results of a tubal pregnancy can be disastrous. An em-

107

bryo that is still partially attached to the wall of the tube may not be expelled for a month or more. Bleeding is intermittent and a mass of blood can form around the end of the tube. This is potentially very serious, because the mass will grow with each bleeding episode until eventually it explodes—usually between the eighth and twelfth weeks. Sometimes the bleeding is so excessive as to be fatal. The tube ruptures with little or no provocation, usually very suddenly.

In both the tubal abortion and the tubal rupture, pain may be severe, although not necessarily. There may also be faintness, nausea, and vomiting. These symptoms result from irritation of the lining of the pelvic cavity, which is particularly sensitive to blood. If bleeding into the pelvic cavity is severe, symptoms of shock—rapid, irregular pulse, pallor, cold, clammy skin, breathing difficulties—will probably occur. If not treated promptly, the patient will die.

Once a tubal pregnancy has been diagnosed, surgery must be performed. And you can't afford to delay too long, because of the risk of fatal bleeding. The surgeon will always try to conserve as much of the tube as possible, especially if you plan to get pregnant again. So let the surgeon know your intentions about future pregnancies.

## HYSTERECTOMY

Hysterectomy is the most commonly performed gynecological operation in the United States—and the most controversial. An estimated 800,000 hysterectomies are performed each year. Yet, one out of three is thought perhaps to be unnecessary. And as the vast majority of women who undergo the procedure are our age, it's important that we all understand the facts. What would you do if, tomorrow, your doctor said you needed to have a hysterectomy?

# What Is It?

Until a few years ago, hysterectomies fell into two categories: a subtotal hysterectomy (removal of the uterus only) and a total hysterectomy (removal of both the uterus and the cervix). Now that the prevalence of cervical cancer is recognized, nearly all hysterectomies include removal of the cervix. For women over forty, a doctor may recommend a bilateral salpingo-oophorectomy. Quite a mouthful! What it means is that along with the uterus and the cervix, the fallopian tubes and the ovaries are also removed, the reason being that older women run an increased risk of developing gynecological ovarian malignancies that would require later surgery.

Lately, there has been a trend to leave the ovaries in place. This shift reflects new concern over osteoporosis, which results from loss of estrogen caused when the ovaries are removed. However, a recent study at George Washington University found that women whose ovaries are left in place run double the risk of dying if they later develop ovarian cancer. In other words, when the ovaries are retained after hysterectomy, these women have an 80 percent ovarian-cancer mortality rate, compared with 40 percent in women who have not had their uterus removed. This finding has prompted the recommendation that we should balance the risk factors associated with developing osteoporosis against this disturbing fact that there's only a 20 percent survival rate among women who develop ovarian cancer after a hysterectomy.

A hysterectomy can be performed in two ways. The most widely used approach is the abdominal hysterectomy, in which an incision is made in the lower abdomen. There is a scar, but in skilled hands it can be an "invisible" one. Most gynecologists use what is called a "bikini cut." The incision is made right above or, if possible, in the pubic hairline and need be no more than four inches long. However, if the surgery involves disease farther up in the abdomen, such as in the ovaries, this low, unobtrusive incision is not usually possible.

109

In the other procedure—a vaginal hysterectomy—the uterus is removed through the vagina. This method is appropriate only in women who have had children, because the ligaments suspending the uterus have relaxed somewhat. But, for a hysterectomy to be performed vaginally, the uterus must be of normal or near-normal size.

Sometimes there's simply no choice in the type of hysterectomy. In severe uterine prolapse—when the uterus bulges into the vagina as a result of stretched ligaments—the vaginal technique must be used. If fibroid tumors have developed in the uterus, the abdominal approach is necessary.

The risk of postoperative infection is higher with vaginal hysterectomy, but recovery is usually quicker and less painful. Whichever the procedure, most women are hospitalized for about seven days. Once they're home, they need lots of rest and should limit their activities for a good six weeks. There's no reason why sexual activity shouldn't continue as before, once you've been given the go-ahead from your doctor and you are comfortable.

## Why the Controversy?

Some of the controversy over hysterectomies exists because many simply don't fall into any clear-cut categories. For example: should a woman with a slight uterine prolapse—not enough to be extremely painful or interfere with bladder function but enough to be bothersome—have a hysterectomy? Many such women will say, "Hey, I'm forty-two, I've got two kids and don't want any more. Why not go ahead with the operation? Who needs periods, anyway?" And how about the argument: "I want to be sterilized, and if I go with a hysterectomy, I'll have the added bonus of not being able to get cancer in my uterus or cervix"?

According to the American College of Obstetricians and Gynecologists, fully 20 percent of all hysterectomies are performed purely as a final solution to the question of contraception. Many such procedures are simply recorded as "uterine prolapse."

But, is hysterectomy a valid contraception option? Surgical sterilization is usually performed by tubal ligation—tying off or cauterizing the fallopian tubes. For all practical purposes, tubal ligation is 100 percent effective, permanent, and relatively simple to perform. However, for many older women, hysterectomy seems more attractive because it also eliminates menstruation and the possibility of two types of cancer that begin to strike when we're in our forties. And those women whose religion forbids out-and-out sterilization (or any other contraceptive method) are quite comfortable with a hysterectomy, "justified" by slight uterine prolapse or excessive bleeding.

Some physicians and some hospitals are disturbed by the idea and may refuse to perform such surgery. Some, however, seem to view it as part of a continuing trend. And it's a trend that stems not from women's ignorance or meek acquiescence to medical pressure but from just the reverse. We women are reading, asking questions, and seeking a variety of opinions. Thanks to the sexual revolution of the sixties, we're now exploring all our options, and as often as not, when we ask for a hysterectomy, it's been a carefully weighed decision.

Of course, many hysterectomies are clearly called for. While every woman who is told she should have a hysterectomy should seek a second opinion, it's useful to know beforehand if your condition warrants that kind of treatment. You'll need a hysterectomy if you have:


- Cancer or precancerous changes in the uterus, ovaries, or fallopian tubes
- Damage to the uterus that cannot be cured by any other means
- Uncontrolled uterine bleeding that cannot be remedied by alternative methods

- Advanced endometriosis that other kinds of treatment have not cured
- Fibroid tumors that are multiple or so large as to be dangerous or impossible to remove with less extensive surgery
- Uterine prolapse which is severe or symptomatic

In general, before heading for the operating room, it's wise to check out the possibility of alternative treatments that are cheaper, less drastic, and safer than surgery. Remember, once the womb is removed, menstruation and childbearing come to an end. There is no reversal possible. Because the outcome is so final, surgery should be performed only when problems cannot be corrected any other way.

## Hysterectomy and the Mind

When it's clear you really must have a hysterectomy, you may go through a period of fear and anxiety. Losing femininity, undergoing premature menopause, becoming unattractive, not being able to have children ever again, or becoming sexually inadequate are some of the more common fears I've heard expressed. It's understandable that for many women hysterectomy can become more of a mental than a physical problem—particularly when self-image has become so inextricably linked with the reproductive organs.

It helps to understand that surgery relieves the problem but does not interfere with sexual functioning. If you have had a total hysterectomy, remember also that it will be much safer for you to have estrogen replacement therapy: there will be no chance of endometrial cancer when you have no uterus!

I find that most women who needed hysterectomies are delighted with their increased energy and freedom from excessive bleeding or backaches. Debbie's experience is typical. At forty-two, she was advised by her gynecologist that the endometriosis that caused her to lose her right ovary ten years ago was getting worse. He recommended removing the left ovary and performing a hysterectomy to prevent recurrent cysts.

"I was scared," she told me. "I thought it would make me dry up and look like an old prune. I'd never enjoy sex again and men wouldn't find me attractive." I introduced Debbie to someone her own age who'd had the operation. "Look at me," Andrea told her. "I look and feel great! And my sex life is better than ever since I don't have to worry about getting pregnant again."

Debbie had the operation and I met with her a few months later. She was dating again and she'd quickly realized that her anxieties were groundless. "I don't know why I was so worried. I really feel good about myself now," she bubbled.

## The Future

With today's enlightened, health-conscious woman, I suspect we are going to see a steady decline in the number of hysterectomies. Sophisticated new surgical techniques will make it increasingly possible to practice far more conservative treatment for those disorders that have traditionally called for hysterectomy. Already a number of medical centers are opening up specifically to offer alternatives. In Los Angeles, for example, there's the new Institute for Reproductive Health, which specializes in the use of microsurgery technology to avoid the need for hysterectomy, except in the case of cancer. Other such centers are opening around the country.

- Fibroid tumors can be surgically removed without hysterectomy.
- Bleeding problems *can* often be treated with hormones, antibiotics, and D and C (dilatation and curettage).
- Pelvic inflammatory disease *can* be effectively treated with antibiotics or limited surgery.

113

- Endometriosis *can* be treated with hormones or limited surgery.

Yes, there *are* alternatives to hysterectomy; but, if hysterectomy is preferred, remember that it is a safe operation and the vast majority of women are thrilled to feel better than they have for years.

## IS SEX BETTER NOW?

For most women entering their fifth decade, life is much easier. We seem to have more direction and we're more content with our lot. Unattainable ambitions that we entertained as teenagers are now forgotten—and so are all those sexual hang-ups! Sex feels good at our age. Our general feeling of confidence and stability makes it so much more enjoyable. And, for most of us, there are no kids around to interrupt!

Regular sexual activity has clear-cut benefits, too. As we approach menopause, an active sex life will actually alleviate many problems that have been associated with the "change of life." San Francisco State University researchers found a direct correlation between a declining frequency of intercourse and an increase in hot flashes, irregular menstrual cycles, and declining estrogen levels.

### Masturbation

Masturbation is also thought to have similar health benefits for women our age. Gone are the days when masturbation was believed to cause mental retardation! Most women are able to achieve orgasm through this technique. It's a completely natural form of sexual expression, with exactly the same body responses that occur with intercourse—increased heart rate, breathing, and muscle tension.

Some sex therapists encourage masturbation as an important part of therapy for women who have difficulty reaching orgasm during intercourse. With masturbation, we can increase our awareness of our own sexuality and better understand what it takes to achieve orgasm—then pass that information on to our partner so that he can provide effective stimulation.

An active sex life keeps the vagina healthy and well toned. If the vagina is not used for extended periods it will begin to atrophy, just like the muscles of the arms and legs if they are not exercised. Many women who have for one reason or another steered away from sex, say for a year or more, find that the vagina has shrunk from lack of use and that when they resume intercourse, it is often painful and sometimes near impossible to achieve penetration. When I discover that a patient is in a situation of celibacy, I tell her it's all right to turn to masturbation—for her health's sake. Masturbation serves a beneficial purpose when intercourse is not available on a regular basis.

Yes, sex at forty feels great! And there's no reason why it shouldn't get better. . . .

# 5

# The New Woman

One undeniable fact for most of us is that we will enter the next decade as *new women*!

We must all pass through "the change of life." For many of us the most disturbing aspect about menopause is not knowing what to expect. And much of what we hear may be old wives' tales. It's unfortunate, but in our culture we tend to dwell on the bizarre and unusual and often overlook the positive side of a life-changing event.

## THE CHANGE OF LIFE

Menopause can open exciting new doors for most of us if only we take the time out to sit down and think of the positive aspects of this inevitable new development in our lives. Don't view menopause as an end to your womanhood, a termination of sexuality, because, if anything, it can mean a rekindling of passion and desire, freed as we are from worries that may have been holding us back for most of our reproductive years. It's

116

a time to let inhibitions fly and wholeheartedly embrace a new sense of freedom and awareness. Mostly, it's a time to take stock of what we can do with our new bodies.

There used to be a strange sort of secrecy about menopause. It wasn't something we women openly talked about, so it's hardly surprising that so many myths abound about the change of life, blaming it for just about everything. Now that it is discussed more between friends and featured prominently in magazines, women may regain their equilibrium in this new phase of life without apprehension.

And with the advent of the latest hormonal-replacement therapies, there is little reason for any woman to approach menopause with anything but the warm confidence that wondrous changes are about to take place.

## When?

Most women will experience menopause between forty-five and fifty-five, though some will have normal menstrual cycles into their sixties. On the other hand, about 8 percent of women are known to reach menopause before their forties, with a few going through the change of life in their early thirties. The average age, however, is fifty-one.

Although it's still not clear just how the body figures out when to turn off the hormone flow, we do know for certain that the age at which a woman undergoes menopause is largely controlled by heredity. You can expect to experience menopause at about the same age your mother or grandmother did. Genetic cues have been passed on to you.

According to statistics from the Department of Health and Human Services, 10 percent of all women will have reached menopause by age forty, 20 percent by forty-three, 50 percent by forty-nine, and almost 100 percent by fifty-eight. Of course, women who suffer damage to their ovaries or have them surgically removed will undergo menopause instantly, no matter what their age.

117

## What Is Menopause?

If you want to look at it from an interesting perspective, menopause is simply puberty in reverse. Puberty prepares our bodies for the act of producing and bearing children, while menopause winds us back down again. It is during puberty that our bodies are first flooded with the hormones estrogen and progesterone.

Menopause is literally the moment that menstruation stops altogether. If you still experience irregular menses, then you haven't reached menopause. If you've gone for as long as six consecutive months without a period, you can be assured you have entered menopause—unless cessation has been caused by an illness or physiological dysfunction. You may not, however, be positive that you cannot become pregnant until one full year has passed since your last period. Menopause itself is part of a much longer phase of changes in the female biological process called the climacteric, which may encompass as much as half a woman's natural life. The climacteric can begin when a woman is in her late twenties or thirties, but usually in her forties, as the production of the estrogen hormone begins to taper off. Once the hormone level has dipped to a low that can no longer stimulate the uterine lining, menstruation stops—but the climacteric does not; it may continue for many years after menopause as estrogen levels continue to drop lower and lower.

## Premenopause

This period is exactly what it sounds like. Although not all women will experience premenopausal symptoms, most will for approximately two years before their periods terminate. It is a time for erratic periods; they may be early or late, heavier than usual or lighter, regular or irregular. This, however, is usually quite normal and nothing to worry about. There are some women who will never experience erratic periods. They'll never notice a premenopausal effect; one month they'll have their last period and that will be that. On the other hand, I have seen patients who have experienced erratic periods for ten years or more before finishing altogether. If you begin to notice irregularity in your cycles, then you should make a visit to your doctor. A thorough pelvic examination will reassure you that the irregular periods are due to hormonal changes. This is also a good time to discuss any other problems and to arrange for a mammogram if you have not had one. Doctors would like to be able to predict how your menstrual pattern will be, but we can't. Every woman is different.

## The Changes

As the hormone levels drop and ovulation ceases, your body will undergo some physical changes. First, because they are no longer needed for reproduction, the ovaries and uterus will begin to shrink in size. The glandular tissue in the breasts will also decrease in size, but fatty tissue replaces it. Now the walls of the vagina will become thinner. Here's where you might hit your first difficulty. As the walls thin down, so does the lubrication system (more about this shortly).

The outward shape of your figure will most likely begin to show changes as well. You'll lose some of the fullness in your hips and breasts, and your waist and upper back will take on a little more bulk. And your skin will be less elastic, drier, because of a decrease in oil production, a lessening of the subcutaneous fat, and a decrease in its moisture-holding capacity.

## Hot Flashes

Yes, this is what a lot of the old wives' tales are all about! Some women are known to quake at the very mention of hot flashes, so it's as well to set the record straight here as to what they're all about. Contrary to popular belief, there is no proven

119

link between symptoms and emotional makeup although the flashes may be distracting and the source of considerable misery.

Hot flashes are perhaps the best known of menopausal symptoms; consequently, they're likely to get the worst press. Gynecologists are still not quite sure what chemical changes in the body cause these sporadic flushes of the face, neck, and upper chest. The presently accepted theory is that hot flashes are due to the decline in estrogen levels in the blood which affects the neurons in the hypothalamic center of the brain: the neurotransmitters in this area are gonadotrophic-releasing hormone GrGH and norepinephrine and they stimulate gonadotropin secretion which episodically causes the temperature control mechanism in the hypothalamus to raise the body temperature in an erratic fashion. With total unpredictability, waves of heat course through the upper body, often followed by heavy sweating. Your face may look red, and the perspiration can make you feel chilly afterward. Usually the episode is much more obvious to the person experiencing it than to an outside observer—which, if anything, should make you feel a bit better!

Hot flashes occur most frequently at night. They produce an actual rise in the body temperature and pump the heart rate up by an average of 13 percent. The flashes last about one to five minutes.

Some of my patients have reported hot flashes occurring as often as twenty times a day, but the average is probably four or five a day for most women. A few women may never experience a single hot flash. The best cure for hot flashes is time, simply letting nature take its course. As the body eventually adjusts to the changing hormone levels, the symptoms decrease and eventually disappear.

There are, however, certain triggers that can set off the waves of heat, and they are to be avoided, if possible. Most common are situations that would normally cause slight temperature elevations, such as anxiety, physical stress, emotional stress, exercise, alcohol, and spicy foods. There have been claims that large doses of vitamin E provide significant easing of unwanted menopausal symptoms, but as far as I am aware, this has not been scientifically or clinically proven.

While definitely not hazardous to your health, hot flashes can be uncomfortable. I've known some patients who report waking up in the middle of the night drenched in perspiration; they throw off the bedclothes, feel cold, and consequently find it difficult to return to sleep. Some women complain that hot flashes reduce their concentration at work, and certainly chronic lack of sleep can be a problem. If you know why something is happening, however, and realize that it's not dangerous to your health, then you don't have to become anxious or frightened. The secret to coping with hot flashes is to understand what's going on and go about your daily life the best you can and ignore them, or treat the symptoms as just a simple, minor, pesky irritation and nothing more. Try to enjoy hot flashes on a cold day!

## Other Symptoms

The overstimulated hypothalamus can create other side effects, such as tingling sensations, insomnia, numbness, palpitations, dizziness, and shortness of breath. Taken as a whole, these might be more than a little debilitating; fortunately, it would be rare for them all to hit at the same time. Like hot flashes, they do decrease with time. These symptoms depend on the rate of estrogen decrease. If it is slow and gradual, they may be less pronounced or never appear at all. The more sudden the drop in estrogen, the more intense the symptoms are likely to be; in effect, it all depends on how much of a shock it is to your system. This is why the recent acceptance of estrogen replacement therapy (ERT) has been such a boon to some women as they pass through menopause.

Although ERT will not halt or reverse the process of the climacteric, it has the advantage to many women of smoothing out a few of the wrinkles they may encounter on the way. ERT dosages are relatively small, but they can help to regulate a too-swift drop in estrogen. However, if you are bothered by any of the abovementioned symptoms and do not want to take hormones, your doctor can suggest other, nonhormonal medications. But more about the benefits—and side effects—of treatment later.

## Sexual Desire

"What's going to happen to my sex life now?" This is the question I'm asked the most . . . and the one I can usually answer in a positive way: you've come a long way sexually, so why stop a good thing now? In fact, many women find that their postmenopausal years are the most sexually active of their lives so far. Why? Wouldn't my sexual desire begin to wane as my female reproductive organs deactivate? Not necessarily so. Libido, or sexual desire, is not affected by the physical changes of menopause. Many women actually feel that menopause has freed them from the fear of becoming pregnant. For once in their lives, they feel relaxed and can settle down to getting the most fulfillment and enjoyment they can out of the sexual experience. Women are known to be capable of orgasm up to their eighties!

## Emotions

Some women experience emotional changes during menopause, and, again, this is normal and nothing to fret about. Just worrying about these emotional lows can plunge them even deeper. It's quite natural for a woman to experience depression, irritability, and fatigue when she's hit with a sudden drop in estrogen whether it occurs premenstrually, directly after childbirth, or in menopause. If physical changes during and after menopause are very obvious, this can also add to the depressive state. Other changes are taking place in

122

your life; parents are aging and may die, and your children may leave the nest. It is often very difficult to juggle the stresses and strains of mid-life—but there is also much to rejoice about despite some losses to contend with. The best advice I can give is to view menopause positively as a source of new sexual freedom and an end to your menstrual cycles, which are troublesome for many women, and look on the change of life as your start as *a new woman*.

## ESTROGEN REPLACEMENT THERAPY (ERT)

So, you want to stay vibrant and youthful and live forever. Forget menopause, just take estrogen supplements and stay the same—fool the body into standing still as time marches on! And why not? Who needs the problems of menopause anyway? Estrogen replacement therapy does sound like we've finally found Ponce de Leon's elusive Fountain of Youth . . . or at least that's the way ERT was being touted back in the early 1940s.

Today we know better.

Estrogen was originally hailed as *the* rejuvenation hormone for females when it was first used by physicians to treat menopausal problems in the forties. By the end of the sixties it was being marveled at as a cure-all for just about anything that ailed the female species. And not only would it keep us healthy; it would make us youthful-looking, replace our thinning hair with lustrous new growth and sheen, awaken our tired old dry, wrinkling skin, firm up our sagging breasts, and revitalize our internal organs.

Considering all this medicine-show hype, it's hardly surprising that estrogen prescriptions rose from below 20 million in the late sixties to almost 30 million by 1975. But it was also in that year that the validity and safety of ERT began to be questioned.

123

It was in 1975 that the first of a host of studies came out that linked postmenopausal estrogen therapy to cancer—mainly, cancer of the lining of the uterus. In 1976 the Food and Drug Administration began to clamp down on the handing out of large doses of estrogen supplements. The FDA's warning was this: only the lowest effective dose of estrogen should be used to ease menopausal symptoms, and then only for the briefest of duration. In effect, the government was saying that it might be okay to take tiny doses of the hormone but harmful to continue them, especially if it was being utilized as a postmenopausal rejuvenator. The American College of Obstetricians and Gynecologists supported this view, and in 1977 pharmaceutical companies manufacturing estrogen were required to explain its risks and benefits in leaflets to be inserted in their product packaging.

Today we can take a more balanced view. And we can see that the mid-seventies rush to exorcise estrogen was possibly an overreaction.

Many physicians do now prescribe estrogen supplements for premenopausal, menopausal, and postmenopausal patients if they see that it will relieve problems or benefit them in some way that will outweigh the potential risk of uterine cancer. It is a conscious decision that has to be made by the physician with the full knowledge and cooperation of his or her patient. Having said that, I must caution that estrogen therapy cannot be taken lightly; there are established risks, and these must be weighed against the undisputed benefits of such therapy. Before starting treatment, it is important to have a mammogram to make sure your breasts are normal. It is also an excellent precaution against uterine cancer to have an endometrial biopsy performed (an office procedure) at regular intervals recommended by your doctor.[1]

## The Cancer Connection

It has been shown that the risk of uterine, or endometrial, cancer increases three to sixfold among women who have been given estrogen supplements alone after menopause. However, when estrogen is administered together with progesterone, it is thought to actually be a protection against cancer. Initially, there was great concern that estrogen was linked with an increase in the rates of breast cancer over the past three decades. Fortunately, this fear has not been borne out. There is not a shred of scientific evidence that can directly link breast cancer with estrogen replacement.

I have always felt that the dosage, the method of administering estrogen, and the length of treatment are all key factors in the risk of endometrial cancer. As with any drug, a little may help but a lot may hinder. Because a specific therapeutic amount works wonders, it does not follow that taking more will work greater miracles. A general consensus among physicians today is that one year on the minimum therapeutic dose (and this may vary widely for individuals) is quite safe and that the risk of uterine cancer increases only after two to four years of continuous therapy.

It must be stressed that there is no average dose for treating menopausal symptoms, and your physician is the only person who will be able to gauge exactly what is therapeutic for you. He may have to do this by trial and error at first, prescribing extremely small doses and gradually increasing them until a beneficial effect is found. He may then want to modify these dosages as you progress through time on the hormone.

Another important consideration, as I mentioned above, is how the estrogen supplements are administered. At one time it was believed that the hormone had to be ingested and work "from the inside out," but that no longer holds true. In fact, among my patients I see remarkable success stories when they are prescribed estrogen-based creams to apply to the vagina for curing itching, soreness, and painful intercourse, but more about that in a moment.

The bottom line is one of hope. Fortunately, careful monitoring can catch most estrogen-related cancers in their earliest stages when they are most curable. The effects of estrogen therapy are reversible as soon as therapy stops. Most research indicates that for women susceptible to the estrogen/cancer link, a two-year estrogen-free period will return the risk of cancer back to the previous level.

## The Benefits of Estrogen Supplements After Menopause

There is no doubt that estrogen prevents or reduces the incidence of hot flashes and the vasomotor symptoms of menopause. It will prevent or lessen vaginal atrophy and there is strong evidence to indicate that estrogen may play a major role in preventing or limiting osteoporosis and even heart disease and other disorders.

Not all the facts are in yet on estrogen's remarkable ability to curb osteoporosis, which is responsible for disfiguring so many women in later life. There are some 300,000 spinal-crush injuries and 250,000 hip fractures in the United States each year, 80 percent of which are estimated to be the direct result of this tragic bone-thinning disease.

The difference in bone loss between men and women is dramatic. At any given age, bone mass is greater in men than in women. During the decade after forty, men lose only about 0.5 percent to 0.75 percent of bone mass yearly, while women in the same age range lose it at more than twice that rate, about 1.5 percent to 2 percent annually. And after menopause in some women that rate may approach 3 percent a year for some time.

Numerous studies have shown that supplemental estrogen prevents bone loss in postmenopausal women. According to one study, the incidence of hip fractures was three times lower among a large group of women on estrogen therapy; and another research team found that the risk of hip fracture was reduced by up to 60 percent in women who had been taking estrogen for six years or longer.

The biggest problem with prescribing estrogen therapy to combat and prevent osteoporosis is knowing which women might already be at risk from the disease. Obviously, to prescribe estrogen for all women because of the chance of osteoporosis is not a viable solution, because of the risk of cancer. Neither is it easy to single out specific women and predict that they will suffer from osteoporosis and should therefore be candidates for long-term estrogen therapy. It is a quandary that only you can solve together with your personal physician.[2]

Preventing heart disease is another distinct advantage of estrogen supplements. It is known that until the onset of menopause, women are greatly protected from heart disease by the delicate balance of the estrogen/progesterone ratio and that after menopause that protective shield is lost, as is evidenced by the fact that the incidence of heart attacks among postmenopausal women doubles. (See pages 183–184.)

We've talked about how menopause, far from signaling an end to sexuality, can release the truly liberated woman within you; there's only one real physical problem that could hold you back—vaginal atrophy. I can't think how many times I have to stress to my patients that this condition is quite normal and easy to manage.

In a recent incident a personal friend came to see me for a postmenopausal gynecological checkup, and I noticed immediately that she must have been having problems. Her vagina had shrunk so much in size that I was hardly able to insert the smallest speculum, and then with great difficulty. I had to treat the situation very gently. "Do you have discomfort when you have intercourse?" I asked. My friend looked a little embarrassed. "Oh, I do get some bleeding and pain," said my highly educated and intelligent friend, "but don't we all at our age? It's expected, isn't it?" The answer is *no*, it's not!

There is absolutely no reason why a woman should endure pain when having intercourse these days just because she has been through menopause. Admittedly the decreasing levels of estrogen can have a noticeable effect on the vagina's ability to function sexually, but this can be ameliorated.

After menopause the pH of the vaginal secretions rises, and

this can promote a more ideal breeding ground for unwanted organisms. At the same time, the vaginal epithelium, or surface skin, dries and thins. In a younger woman the layers of cells that build up the vaginal walls will probably number over thirty, but after menopause they can be reduced to a scant, fragile half-dozen layers. The result is an increased susceptibility to irritation, injury, and infection.

These changes will progress with time. The vagina can begin to shrink and lose much of its elasticity, softness, and plumpness. The interior of the vagina may become shorter and more rigid. On the outside, the labia majora become less pronounced, flatter, and lighter in color. This lightening is due to the decrease of blood flowing through the vaginal lips because of the decrease in estrogen. In effect, the vagina is shrinking. The condition is called atrophic vaginitis—not exactly conducive to the pleasures of lovemaking.

The first most noticeable problem post menopause is a distinct lack of lubrication, especially during the preliminaries to intercourse and the start of the act itself. There are glands at the entrance to the vagina, called Bartholin's glands, which provide some lubrication, but this usually occurs during lovemaking. It is this lack of initial lubrication that puts many women off even attempting any penetration at all. The biggest cry I hear from my postmenopausal patients is, "If this is what my sex life's going to be like after the change, then forget it!" The vagina has no lubricating glands; it relies on a "sweating" effect brought on by a rapid increase of blood flow to the tissues of the vagina. During our younger years, the arousal stage is quite swift and the vagina can be fully lubricated in a matter of twenty to thirty seconds. As we approach menopause, the foreplay necessary to "get the juices flowing" may have to be longer. Without the estrogen levels that promote increased blood flow to the vagina, the lubricating response decreases and eventually is lost altogether.

This is where topical estrogen creams come in. By applying these creams onto and around the vagina and massaging them

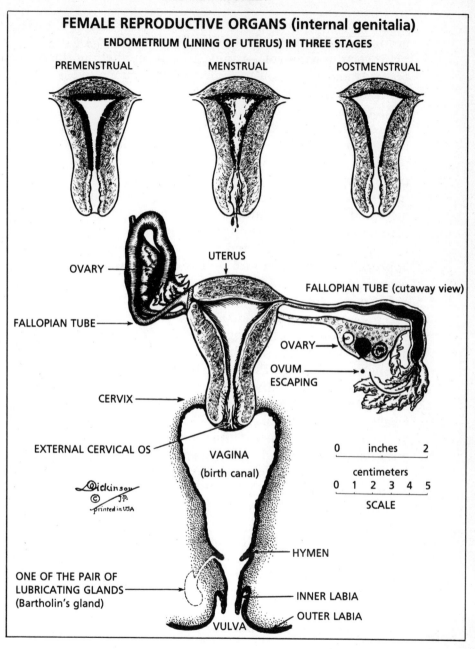

**FEMALE REPRODUCTIVE ORGANS (internal genitalia)**

**ENDOMETRIUM (LINING OF UTERUS) IN THREE STAGES**

PREMENSTRUAL        MENSTRUAL        POSTMENSTRUAL

OVARY

UTERUS

FALLOPIAN TUBE (cutaway view)

FALLOPIAN TUBE

OVARY

OVUM ESCAPING

CERVIX

EXTERNAL CERVICAL OS

VAGINA (birth cal)

0    inches    2

centimeters

0  1  2  3  4  5

SCALE

HYMEN

ONE OF THE PAIR OF LUBRICATING GLANDS (Bartholin's gland)

INNER LABIA

OUTER LABIA

VULVA

129

in, you resupply the estrogen hormone directly to where it is needed—and it can work miracles. Vaginal dryness is relieved, pH reverts to its normal acidity, and the epithelium thickens, becomes more resistant to injury and infection, and is better lubricated. In effect, you are able to rejuvenate your own vagina with no fuss or trouble.

I regularly prescribe estrogen creams for postmenopausal women, as I did for my friend. She was like many of my patients, extremely skeptical that it would work. Studies of postmenopausal women between the ages of fifty and seventy have indicated that the flow of blood to the vagina is greatly increased by the stimulating effect of local application of supplemental estrogen. After just one month of therapy, the improved blood flow resulted in levels of vaginal fluids that approached those of a group of women between the ages of twenty and forty.

If you suffer from premenopausal vaginal problems, or you've been through menopause, do yourself a favor and consider the wonders of estrogen cream. Don't forget, you are applying this directly to where it's needed and not ingesting it long-term through the entire body. Although I stress this, I don't mean it to lull you into a false sense of security. The American Medical Association recently pointed out that two locally effective vaginal creams—Estrace and Premarin—have been shown to be absorbed into the bloodstream. Indeed, long-term daily use revealed estrogen levels in the blood approaching those of oral estrogen replacement therapies. Because the hormone is absorbed into the bloodstream from the vaginal tissues, the overall dosage is quite erratic as it is not an exactly measured dose like a pill taken orally, and rates of absorption may vary. Last year the FDA approved the use of a skin patch (or transdermal application) of estrogen. The rate of absorption seems to be very even, and the great advantage is that the hormone does not have to be processed through the liver, which reduces the possibility of certain side effects. Other drugs, such as scopolamine for travel sickness and nitroglycerine for angina, work beautifully in this way, so there's a good chance that this will be the best way to take estrogen in the future—through your skin!

However, don't expect everything to happen overnight. It may take a month or two before you start noticing an improvement.

If vaginal dryness still interferes with the comfort of intercourse, don't be shy: turn to self-lubrication with gels like K-Y, Surgilube, or those produced especially for intercourse. Petroleum-based products, like Vaseline, should not be used as lubricants. Many women are sensitive to petroleum bases; also, as they are not water solvent, they are difficult to remove. For many women, a good dab of gel at the opening of the vagina will be sufficient to allow the penis to enter comfortably.

## Side Effects

For some women, there are undesirable side effects associated with estrogen therapy, but these are few and mild. They include: swollen breasts, vaginal discharge, irritability, headaches, nausea, elevated blood pressure, and weight gain. Women who take both estrogen and progesterone sometimes notice vaginal bleeding at the end of each month, though this should be lighter than a regular period.

## Toward a New Freedom

So, now you can forget all the old wives' tales you heard about the change of life, because I've just given you the thoroughly modern woman's view on menopause. Throw away those old fears and trepidations and take a fresh new look at the bonuses being offered during the next decade. It's a future of new freedoms through change for you to enjoy as a new woman!

# 6

# Common Problems

You've probably been aware that some relatively new buzz-words have crept into the everyday vocabulary of health problems over the past few years. You have certainly heard and read of PMS (premenstrual syndrome), TSS (toxic shock syndrome), PID (pelvic inflammatory disease), and UTI (urinary tract infection). They may sound like a bewildering array of letters and problems, but they all have one thing in common: these conditions are strictly for women only. They are, shall we say, the crosses we have to bear as females.

But, while these disease entities may plague us, the *good* news is: the odds are in our favor that we'll live to a ripe old age. American women are healthier and surviving longer than their mothers and grandmothers. And we're getting better at it all the time.

By the twenty-first century (not much more than a decade away, ladies), the life expectancy for a woman will be 81.05 years. At present, a girl born today can anticipate attaining the grand old age of 77.53 years. Compare that with the average life expectancy of a woman born in 1900 (49.7 years) and you can easily see that we've made great strides since just the beginning of this century.

What's causing our new longevity? First, the continual progress of modern medicine provides us with successful treatment for most infectious diseases, as well as for many metabolic, endocrinological, gastrointestinal, and hereditary disorders, while sophisticated anesthesia and surgical techniques make operations safer than ever before. Second, very simply, we women have assumed more control over our health, we're better educated about our bodies, and we're not kept in the dark as much as we used to be. While the wife and mother might have been given a pat on the back by the paternalistic male physician of the past, today the educated woman of the eighties is not only a force but also a mind to reckon with. We have demanded attention to our bodies; we've insisted on answers, and now we've got most of them. Third, we're eating smarter today, we exercise more, and generally we take far better care of ourselves than did the generations before us. The big payoff is that we are preventing and fighting disease like never before.

Heart disease is the number-one killer in this country, but although cardiovascular diseases still cause over 50 percent of deaths among women today, the death rate from heart attack has actually dropped 38 percent in the last two decades. Recognizing the threat posed by high blood pressure and seeking early treatment has had a strong impact on women's lives. So has watching our weight and cholesterol, controlling our intake of salt, getting more exercise, and avoiding stress.

Although cancer is still our biggest killer, especially among women between thirty-five and fifty-five, the death rate from cancer of the reproductive organs and bladder has substantially decreased. On the negative side, the percentage of deaths from breast cancer has remained approximately the same since the late forties, and as more women than ever before are smoking today, the death rate for lung cancer among us has doubled since 1970.

But let's not look on the gloomy side. While there are obvious health insurance policies we can take out, like quitting smoking, sticking to an exercise program, and further improving our dietary habits, there are other less obvious pathways to good health.

## THE VALUE OF PERSONAL AND FAMILY HISTORY

Learning as much as we can about our family health history is possibly the single most important preventive step we can take against ill health and disease at this stage in our lives. Why? Because we may have inherited genes from our family tree that make us more apt to develop certain illnesses which could be prevented or attenuated if, knowing about them early enough, we change our diet or lifestyle or avoid certain precipitating factors. Our grandmothers may still be around, but possibly not for long. Many of us will still have the benefit of a mother to consult about family history, but as we all get older, memories get shakier and there's a lot that might be missed if we don't act.

The first thing I advise a new patient who may be approaching or is in her forties is to start compiling a personal medical history of herself, her family, and especially her maternal female ancestors whenever possible. Whether you realize it now or not, this may be one of the most useful health guides you can pass on to your own daughters and granddaughters.

Begin a log, and start by recording your own childhood diseases, inoculations, developmental problems, or any conditions you have had since birth. Next, list major illnesses and hospital stays. Try to recall the names of the hospitals, attending physicians, and specific diagnostic tests and procedures you underwent. Pay particular attention to the type of surgery you had, the type of anesthesia, any complications—

including allergies to foods and drugs—and list all the drugs that were prescribed for you. Have you ever had hay fever, eczema, asthma, or wheezing?

Let's go to your gynecological history now. Record your first onset of menstruation and any problems you may have experienced up to date. Record the methods of birth control you have used, when you may have switched to the Pill and which brands you have taken. List your pregnancies and outcomes, including natural births, C-sections, difficult deliveries, and miscarriages. Although I wouldn't expect any of you to have undergone menopause yet, in a few rare cases this can happen. If you have experienced any menopausal symptoms, make a careful note of them, too.

What's your occupational and social history? These can be valuable indicators of stress-related problems, to which so many illness and disease states seem to be linked today. For your job history, include positions, working hours, job-related injuries, and exposure to potentially hazardous materials. On the social side, list your sports activities, exercise programs you follow regularly, nutrition, and dietary habits. Do yourself a big favor and honestly record your intake of alcohol and any other "social" drugs. If you smoke, jot down how many cigarettes a day and how long you have been smoking.

Now for the family history and possible new sources of clues to your present health and red flags for what may be to come. Write down the ages and health of your parents, grandparents, brothers, sisters, and other close relatives. If any of them are dead, indicate cause of death. Heart disease, cancer, arthritis, diabetes, and hypertension are notorious for running in families. The farther back you can go, the better. If you cannot rely on memory alone, don't forget that most families usually have an old box stashed away somewhere in the attic that contains old newspaper clippings about family history, important events, birth certificates, and, most importantly, death certificates. As morbid as it may sound, autopsy reports can carry an untold wealth of medical information that may reflect directly on yourself. If you feel you don't have enough information about what has happened to you, it is possible to write to doctors or hospitals where you were treated, even if it was years ago.

The best time to start collecting this invaluable information is *now*. And remember, continually keep updating your records as any significant health changes take place in your life or in the lives of your relatives.

## THE IMPORTANCE OF PHYSICALS

Pap smears, mammograms, and regular physical exams are your best line of defense against the problems that plague us women the most.

And age is the key factor to protection and life extension when it comes to the tests-that-save. What may be appropriate for a woman in her twenties and thirties is not so for the woman of forty.

Most medical practitioners will agree that a complete physical conducted every year is not cost-effective for the general population, although an annual visit to discuss problems and have a breast examination is ideal. If you undergo the standard battery of tests too frequently, you can find yourself racking up hundreds of dollars in medical expenses. Today, periodic screening tests based on age are a far more concrete way to insure good health and nip any problems in the bud.

The following is a checklist of tests, based on the recommendations of the American Academy of Family Practice, which I advise all my patients to follow.

Beginning at age forty:

- A complete general physical examination, including laboratory tests, blood count, urinalysis, hearing and vision tests, EKG, and chest X ray. This should be repeated every five years until the age of sixty. Over sixty,

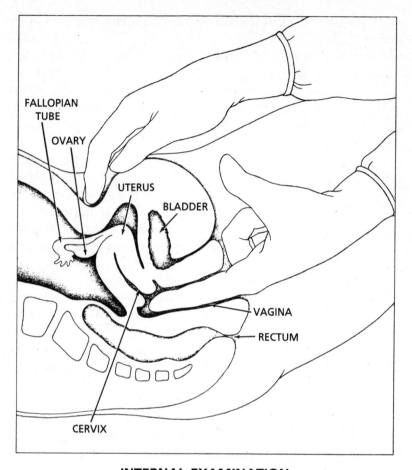

FALLOPIAN TUBE
OVARY
UTERUS
BLADDER
VAGINA
RECTUM
CERVIX

## INTERNAL EXAMINATION

This is how your gynecologist conducts a pelvic examination. Utilizing pressure and feeling internal organs, many common problems can be easily detected. *The National Cancer Institute* these checkups should be stepped up to once every two years.

- Pelvic exam and Pap test should have been conducted every one to two years until the age of forty. You can ease off these a little now and make them every two years unless you are in a high-risk group for cervical cancer (see page 214). After the age of sixty you will not need to have them done so often.
- Breast examination. This should have been performed annually and hopefully you have been doing your breast self-examination also. You should continue with an annual breast examination; if you are at high risk for breast cancer, you should be checked more frequently. Your blood pressure will be taken also at the visit and a check can be kept on your weight.
- Mammography for breast cancer. Current recommendations include a baseline study between thirty-five and forty, then mammograms every one to two years from forty to fifty, when they should begin to be performed annually. Only a mammogram can pick up a very early cancer that cannot be felt on breast examination (see page 204.)
- Stool test for blood and sigmoidoscopy for colon cancer. The stool test should start at age forty (earlier if you have a positive family history) and the sigmoidoscopy should be performed every three to five years (more frequently if you are at high risk; see page 211).
- Endometrial biopsy, a suction test to look for cancer of the uterine lining, should be done for any irregular bleeding or if you are on ERT (see pages 123 and 216).

Remember, there are special tests you should take if you are planning children or intending to have more. A test for German-measles immunity is imperative. And a complete obstetrical examination should be conducted during the first trimester of pregnancy. This should include blood counts, blood and Rh type, syphilis test, urinalysis, and Pap tests.

# COMMON PROBLEMS

By far the best weapon a woman has in her personal health arsenal is a thorough understanding of the problems she may face. At no time in your life may it be more important than now. Not every one of the following problems hits directly in the forties. Some have broad age ranges, so we would be remiss to ignore them.

It's not my intention to baffle you with the medical complexities of these conditions but to supply you with an idea of what to expect and when, how to cope, and what latest treatments are available.

# PREMENSTRUAL SYNDROME (PMS)

One way of keeping premenstrual syndrome in perspective is remembering that once we hit our forties, it won't be with us much longer. But, in the meantime, you don't necessarily have to suffer. Latest research indicates that there are a number of steps you can take to alleviate the physical and mental anguish of PMS.

What exactly is PMS? Well, if you suffer from it regularly, you're likely to describe it as the worst scourge ever inflicted upon the female gender. Generations of PMS sufferers have been ignored; your mother, grandmother, and great-grandmother may have been PMS sufferers, but they probably kept quiet about it, since there was very little understanding or sympathy for women who got monthly bouts of unexplainable irritability and moodiness.

PMS has recently been described as one of the most critical women's health issues in the United States. In Great Britain,

PMS has been upheld as a legitimate defense in at least two murder trials of women who unexplainably turned homicidal. France now accepts the problem as legitimate grounds for a plea of temporary insanity. We've come a long way in recognizing PMS as a bona-fide physical problem faced by some women and not just the product of the female psyche.

It's now widely accepted that PMS is caused by a hormonal imbalance with resulting water retention. From two to fourteen days before our periods, many of us begin to feel a distinct change. We feel bloated, our breasts become tender and sore, and our skin breaks out. We get headaches and gain weight. Other accompanying symptoms include feeling listless, nervous, depressed, restless, tense, and sometimes quite agitated. For some women, it might feel very similar to being at war with the entire rest of the world. We doctors can now attribute some fifty or so symptoms that can be directly traced back to what we call PMS.

These symptoms stay pretty constant each month for PMS sufferers. Some of us actually adapt our life-styles to cope with them. We might forego a romantic candle-lit dinner or a welcome trip to the theater or movies, preferring to hang around the house in misery rather than be seen at our worst. We learn to compensate. Some women may sleep more, eat more, and retire more into themselves; it's a kind of self-preservation. We learn to do things like putting on a brave face at work, gritting our teeth, and grinning and bearing it, knowing, thank goodness, that it won't last more than a few days at the most. Strangely, there is a very tiny minority of PMS sufferers who actually feel more vibrant and energized. They are, however, very much the exception to the rule.

After all is said and done, none of these methods of handling PMS effects a cure. There is no cure!

## Beating the PMS Blues and Blahs

While there may be no cure, we have made significant progress in finding alternative methods to cope with PMS. Altering the diet and preventing water retention, it has been shown, greatly ameliorate the symptoms felt by many women. We now know that the natural amino acid tryptophan is integral to maintaining sufficient levels of a brain chemical called serotonin, a neurotransmitter that controls appetite, sleep, and, yes, pain and depression—two prominent factors in PMS.

New studies indicate that levels of free (available) tryptophan in the blood can take a dip some days prior to menstruation. (It's theoretically possible that the decline in tryptophan may be due to significant shifts in hormone levels.) Boosting these levels by dietary means during the PMS days may greatly help to alleviate many sufferers' symptoms.

Tryptophan is found in all protein foods, but that doesn't necessarily mean that eating huge steaks and burgers is going to raise blood tryptophan levels; in fact, conversely, it may have the opposite effect. In a unique series of chemical changes within the body, tryptophan's conversion to serotonin in the brain is actually helped along by chemicals found in carbohydrates. A little bit of protein goes a long way in supplying tryptophan, but a healthy portion of carbohydrates eaten at the same time will greatly enhance the tryptophan potential. The best way to capitalize on tryptophan during those blah days is to eat a reduced-protein, low-fat, high-carbohydrate diet (see Chapter 8 for more details).

Vitamin $B_6$ (pyridoxine) has also been found to bring relief from PMS symptoms. Recently it was discovered that levels of the vitamin drop immediately prior to menstruation and doctors believe that there is a definite link between a lack of $B_6$ and premenstrual depression. There's yet another fascinating connection here: $B_6$ also plays a crucial chemical role in maintaining sufficient levels of tryptophan. Surprising?

If you add tryptophan and $B_6$ as individual daily supplements to your diet, or take a daily multivitamin that supplies each, you are assured of an adequate supply of both nutrients. Combine that with good balanced eating—less on the burgers and heavier on the potatoes and pastas—and you may have found a purely natural way to curb your PMS symptoms.

141

Prevention of water retention is obviously the key to minimizing PMS symptoms. If you have tried dietary measures to increase your tryptophan and B$_6$ levels for one or two cycles without relief then it's time to consider ways to prevent this water build-up in your body. I tell my patients that while fluid retention is uncomfortable in your breasts and abdomen where the tissues are soft and elastic and can swell and shrink easily, just a little extra water in your brain (enclosed by your hard bony skull) creates relatively more pressure and makes you irritable, headachey, jumpy, and depressed.

So, to prevent fluid buildup you should take less in and stay away from anything that helps water stay in your body. While it is generally thought healthy to drink lots of water daily to keep your body well hydrated, your urine not concentrated, and your intestinal contents softer, this does *not* apply to PMS sufferers. Even if you feel thirsty before menstruation drink just a sip or two of water; don't indulge your thirst. Two items in our diet cause fluid to stay in the tissues rather than be passed quickly out in the urine: salt and caffeine. Caffeine restriction, for example, minimizes discomfort from, and the size of, breast cysts and all surgeons suggest women with cystic breasts eliminate caffeine in their diet before they attempt to treat the cysts by aspirating fluid with a needle. Often there is great improvement on restricting coffee, tea, chocolate, caffeinated sodas and over-the-counter medications containing caffeine. So it makes sense premenstrually to eliminate caffeine from your diet. If you cut down salt in the second half of your cycle (and many women crave salty foods then) it will reduce fluid retention as sodium is known to keep water in the tissues of the body. Remember how people with high blood pressure are told to keep on a low-sodium diet? It is for this reason: more water is excreted by the kidneys if the sodium content of the diet is reduced. So try this also for PMS: avoid salty foods such as ham, bacon, cold cuts, canned soups and vegetables, potato chips, pickles, ketchup, and saltines. Most women find it works if they really make an effort to reduce salt and caffeine: simple, inexpensive ways of coping with PMS!

If you still have problems then the judicious use of mild diuretics prescribed by your doctor to use premenstrually should give you relief. At the University of Connecticut Health Center in Farmington, doctors found that 80 percent of a group of PMS sufferers who took spironolactone, a potassium-sparing diuretic, were recorded as having significant relief from PMS symptoms. The drug seems to work by blocking production of a hormone which is linked to the mood swings, bloating, and tenderness associated with PMS. Dr. Carlos Soto-Albors, who headed the study, reports that spironolactone was particularly successful in relieving depression and crying spells.

I much prefer that women handle their PMS and stay in control of their bodies by choosing a careful diet, as I've just outlined, getting daily exercise, and limiting caffeine and salt intake for the crucial two weeks of their cycle. It can make an enormous difference.

## TOXIC SHOCK SYNDROME (TSS)

Because toxic shock syndrome can strike women of any age at any time, the possibility of encountering it should not be ignored. However, the chances against contracting it are in your favor. A woman in her forties is more likely to have built up an immunity to the microorganism, *Staphylococcus aureus,* that is thought to precipitate TSS. Any woman of menstruating age is particularly vulnerable to the condition. And as yet, nobody is absolutely sure how one "catches" the bacterium, though many studies link it directly to tampon use.

There's much speculation as to the tampon's instrumental role in TSS, but most likely a combination of factors is responsible. For instance, plastic applicators used to insert tampons can scratch the walls of the vagina and cause micro-lacerations, minute cuts that can be an open door for the toxin to get into

143

the bloodstream. Another possibility is that we may inadvertently transfer the bacterium from our fingers when inserting a tampon. A third determining factor may be the new super-absorbent chemicals used in tampons, which can dry out the normally moist vagina, thus damaging the delicate membrane forming its walls and leaving it open to micro-ulcerations and infections.

## Protecting Against TSS

For the mature woman with a lifetime history of using tampons, there should be little cause to fear toxic shock syndrome, because of inbuilt immunity. However, it's as well for us all to recognize the symptoms. Toxic shock strikes suddenly. The first warning may be a sudden wave of dizziness or weakness, followed by vomiting, diarrhea, chills, aching muscles, and a temperature of at least 102 degrees. Other symptoms to be aware of include irritation in the throat, nose, or vagina, headache, inflamed eyes, and a rash that resembles sunburn.

Here's what I advise my patients to do to lower the risk:

- Wash your hands before insertion or removal of a tampon.
- Never wait more than eight hours to change a tampon.
- Avoid using tampons at night or when your menstrual flow is slight.
- Avoid using high absorbancy tampons.
- If you're using a tampon when any of the symptoms appear, remove it at once.
- See your physician immediately if symptoms strike.
- Don't use tampons again if you've experienced the symptoms of TSS previously.

144

# OSTEOPOROSIS

You've no doubt heard a lot about osteoporosis recently. And if you have, no doubt calcium was also mentioned. We'll get to the pros and cons of this essential mineral a little later. The fact is that most mature women are now beginning to sit up and take note of the terrible effects of this disease, especially on the elderly female.

Osteoporosis is not new; it's been around as long as womankind. What has recently made the difference in our awareness of it is the recognition that the older female is far more prone to suffer its debilitating effects than any other segment of the population. The symptoms of osteoporosis include back pain, loss of height, and a disfiguring curvature of the spine known as dowager's hump.

Should we fear it in our forties? The simple answer is no. But what we should be doing now is taking preventive measures to ensure that it never catches up with us.

## What Is It?

Osteoporosis is a thinning of the density of the bone matrix—the internal scaffolding that provides the strength and support for every bone in your body. The insides of bones are a honeycomb of supporting structures that determine their tremendous strength and even flexibility. If that bone mass begins to erode, the bone is especially prone to breaks. The same stress which would cause a simple hairline fracture in the bone of a young woman would cause a complete fracture in an osteoporosis victim. And the bigger and longer the bone, the more weight the bone mass has to carry; thus, the more susceptible it will be to breakage. For the woman severely afflicted with osteoporosis, a simple tap on the shin can result in a major fracture.

## Whom Does It Affect?

Well, us, period. To begin with, women's bones are about 30 percent smaller than men's, meaning we may be carrying a similar load on a lighter subframe. At the onset of menopause, we begin losing bone mass at an accelerated rate due to the drop in the protective effect of estrogen, making us more than eight times more prone to the disease than men.

In a single year, osteoporosis treatment costs upward of $4 billion, and the number of women at risk is beginning to grow. There's a simple reason for this: in 1980, 40 percent of American women were over forty; by the year 2000, that figure is expected to rise to 50 percent, or half the female population.

Osteoporosis has had an enormous epidemiological impact on us women; it affects over 10 million of us, including 26 percent of all women over sixty. So, for the woman of the fifth decade, it is clear that the seeds may already be sown.

## Risk Factors

To fight osteoporosis effectively, we must be able to recognize it long before symptoms and irreversible damage can occur. High-risk women are Caucasians with fair complexions, slight builds, sedentary habits, premature or surgical menopause, and family history of the disease. Many researchers suggest that excessive consumption of cigarettes, alcohol, and caffeine are also factors.

There is also a condition known as premature osteoporosis. Women who engage in extended strenuous exercise, such as running, often stop having menstrual periods. Research now indicates that prolonged amenorrhea (lack of periods) can result in premature osteoporosis. At the University of California, San Francisco, radiologists noted a significant loss of bone density in women who had stopped menstruating from one to twenty-two years earlier. Women who experience a cessation of their periods due to endocrine disorders run the same risk.[1]

## A Cure: The Great Calcium Hype

Now that your calcium pills have found their special niche in the medicine cabinet, here's the not-so-good news: reliance on them alone to ward off osteoporosis is creating a false sense of security. And overuse of calcium supplements may even pose a threat to your health.

We are already consuming ten times more calcium than we once did. Once the medical profession announced the possible calcium/osteoporosis link, the vitamin and mineral manufacturers were fast to catch on that an exploding new market was opening up for them. In fact, what was once a $17-million business has now become a $200-million windfall for calcium-supplement manufacturers.

I don't doubt the need for calcium in the fight against osteoporosis, especially as it's abundantly clear that we need more of this mineral than was previously believed; but pill-popping as a means of boosting calcium levels in the bones is fraught with controversy—and risk. Indiscriminate self-medication with calcium supplements can put a few of us in danger of developing hypercalcemia (abnormally high calcium levels found in the blood) and kidney stones.

The truth is that only two out of some fifteen major studies support the beneficial effect of calcium supplements in the war against osteoporosis. What has been demonstrated beyond any doubt is that women who have osteoporosis lack calcium in their natural diets. And it's a fact that calcium in pill form is not absorbed as well as the calcium we receive through our foods.

## Sensible Prevention

Eating foods that have a high calcium content is about the best way to take out an insurance policy against osteoporosis.

The Recommended Dietary Allowance for calcium is eight hundred milligrams per day; one thousand to fifteen hundred milligrams for postmenopausal, pregnant, and nursing women. Milk and milk products are the best sources of dietary calcium. A cup of milk—whole, skim, or 99 percent fat free—provides three hundred milligrams. Other sources rich in calcium include navy and pinto beans, tofu, collard greens, broccoli, kale, almonds, salmon, and sardines with the soft bones intact.

I strongly recommend that you take no more than half the daily requirements in supplement form. Try to get into the habit of good nutrition and get most of your required calcium

**MEAN CALCIUM INTAKE (mg)**

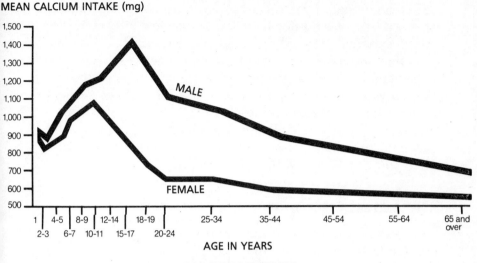

## CALCIUM INTAKE

This diagram illustrates the decline in female calcium intake with age and how vitally important it may be to use calcium supplements. *Marion Laboratories Inc.*

from the foods you eat each day. Do not wait for menopause symptoms to start—begin now! Most women's diets are calcium-deficient from adolescence, so changing your calcium intake now will be very beneficial.

Estrogen replacement therapy (ERT), mainly prescribed for menopausal and postmenopausal women, has been shown to reduce greatly the risk of calcium deficiency. If you are experiencing early menopausal signs, this may be the avenue you might also want to follow. Read the section on ERT in Chapter 5 for the pros and cons about this form of treatment and consult with your physician.

Exercise is yet another way to combat osteoporosis. It is known that weight-bearing exercise, such as tennis or jogging strengthens bones in younger people. To see how it affected the mature woman, researchers at the University of North

Carolina compared women who played tennis a few times a week with those who normally led an inactive life. The fifty-five-to-sixty-five-year-old tennis players had much more bone mass than sedentary women of the same age.

Remember I said *weight-bearing* exercise helps keep the calcium in your bones. Swimming and bicycling, while excellent for your heart, lungs, and muscle tone, are not useful in preventing osteoporosis. Walking, running, dancing, tennis, and golf are better choices for this purpose. So consider your bones when you choose a new form of exercise.

## The Latest Osteoporosis Test

A new, highly accurate, inexpensive test can detect osteoporosis early enough for the disease to be reversed. "It's a major advance that will help millions of Americans, particularly postmenopausal women," reports Martin Sandler, M.D., associate professor of radiology and medicine at Vanderbilt University Medical Center in Nashville.

Presently, eight hundred hospitals and doctors' offices are performing the test at an average cost to the patient of $125, although this price should drop significantly as the devices become more widely used over the next year or so. Until now there has not been a highly sensitive test that could record bone thinning in its earliest stages. But the new test, using dual-photon absorptiometry (DPA), can screen postmenopausal women and other high-risk groups in as little as fifteen minutes. The patient lies on a table, and a computerized scanner—similar to a sophisticated X-ray machine—sends a narrow radiation beam through the body and into the bones. The amount of radiation is significantly less than that of a conventional chest X ray. Data about the density of the bones is then fed into a computer that calculates the mineral composition in terms of grams per square centimeter. This figure is then compared with those for average bone density of disease-free individuals of the same age. The test is so accurate that physicians are able to spot a mere 3 percent drop in bone mass.

Dr. Sandler, who has tested more than five thousand patients as part of his research, points out that all bones can be examined, and the test is the first capable of measuring bone mass in the hip, site of some of the most common and serious fractures. For postmenopausal women, DPA is an excellent screening test for osteoporosis. "I recommend every woman to have the test within two years of finishing menopause, because the best treatment results are obtained when osteoporosis is detected less than two years after onset," says Dr. Sandler. "Women who show signs of the disease should have follow-up tests every year to assess the response to therapy. Those who are initially disease-free should probably be screened every two or three years."

DPA is reported to be safe, painless, and an excellent choice of diagnosis for those in high-risk categories, such as women who are taking medications that can rob the bones of calcium, or those with kidney disease and thyroid problems.

The choice is yours. Preventing osteoporosis should be part of every woman's daily routine. As women are living longer than ever, it's even more important that their bones be strong enough to meet the demands of those golden years. A few ounces of prevention at this stage in our lives can keep our bones healthy.


# ARTHRITIS

Although arthritis can strike at any age, its onset is most common in women between their thirties and fifties. And the disease afflicts three times more women than men. More than 40 million Americans presently suffer from arthritis, and new cases are occurring at a rate of one million a year.

The word *arthritis*, which quite literally means inflammation of the joint, describes not just one disease but a multitude of complaints. There are about one hundred varieties of painful and sometimes crippling conditions that fall under the umbrella of "arthritis," the two most common being osteoarthritis and rheumatoid arthritis.

Osteoarthritis mainly affects the woman who is fifty or older. Its first telltale signs are stiffness and pain in one or more joints, usually the larger weight-bearing joints, like the hips and knees, but also joints that are well worked, like those of the fingers and thumbs, toes, and neck. It causes a loss of elasticity in the tissues, called cartilage, that cushion the bone in the joints. Eventually sections of the cartilage can wear away, leaving the bone exposed and even more vulnerable to wear and tear. Clearly, being overweight will make the symptoms worse and degenerative changes in the weight-bearing joints happen sooner. The good news about osteoarthritis, as if there could be any, is that few victims suffer any seriously debilitating symptoms.

Rheumatoid arthritis, on the other hand, is a crippling disease. This occurs when the lining of the joints, called the synovial membrane, becomes inflamed. We physicians are not even sure why this disease strikes, although the latest thinking is that it is closely connected with the immune system and may actually be caused by an immune-system dysfunction. We do know that it can cause great pain and stiffness in the joints most often affected: the knuckles, wrists, knees, elbows, and shoulders.


## Treatment

We do not yet have the knowledge to cure arthritis, so until we do, the best approach is treatment that will control the advance of the disease and help ease the painful symptoms. Aspirin is an excellent first choice of drug to give symptomatic relief. It is inexpensive, readily available, usually helpful and relatively nontoxic. Care must be taken because it can cause gastrointestinal irritation and bleeding but when taken with an antacid this is usually avoided. Aspirin is better taken continually rather than intermittently.

The relatively new pain-relieving nonsteroidal anti-inflammatory drugs (NSAIDs) have been a boon to sufferers from arthritis. More long-acting than aspirin, a bedtime dose will minimize morning stiffness and pain. The NSAIDs also cause gastric upset and can be toxic to the kidneys and have neurological side effects: twenty-five times more costly than aspirin, they should be prescribed and the dose regulated by your physician. It is reassuring to know that research continues on arthritis and its prevention and treatment. New drugs are constantly coming on the market. Prolonged use of potent drugs such as steroids, while having a desirable effect in reducing pain and stiffness, may cause a bloated appearance due to buildup of fatty tissue especially on the face and trunk. Steroids are also known to suppress the immune system—which, especially considering the possible cause of rheumatoid arthritis, is a Catch-22 situation.

The best way to tackle arthritis is through rest, aspirin or a physician-prescribed nonsteroidal anti-inflammatory drug, weight loss, a calcium-rich diet, and sex. . . . Yes, I said sex!

According to the Arthritis Foundation, recent studies indicate that sex in moderation (whatever they mean by that!) temporarily relieves the pain of arthritis. We've always believed that sex can be a good tonic, but now there is solid scientific evidence to show its benefits in fighting pain. Many of my patients have reported, mostly as a humorous aside, that they notice relief from their aches and pains for long periods after having sex. Researchers now speculate that the sex act releases a shot of the body's own natural painkillers, brain chemicals called endorphins. In studies, women have reported being desensitized from arthritis pain for as long as three hours—and in a few cases as long as a day—after a rousing sexual escapade. As an added benefit, active sex is a good form of physical therapy.

So what do those of us who are presently unattached, in

153

between, still searching, or saving ourselves for Mr. Right do? The simple, straightforward answer is, masturbation. It is the act of arousal and fulfillment that releases those important endorphins, whether it's performed by one or two. If you're not active with a regular partner, this is something for you to consider.

Here's an interesting sidelight that links well with sex: for those of you still interested, getting pregnant also appears to have a soothing effect on arthritis. Nature may actually have provided pregnant women with a special arthritis remedy. For years women with rheumatoid arthritis have reported a dramatic decrease in pain once they became pregnant. Pregnant women have been found to have a high blood concentration of a protein substance called pregnancy alpha-glycoprotein (PAG), which is currently thought to be responsible for pain relief in pregnancy. And it raises the possibility of an all-natural drug to fight arthritis. PAG is thought to work by suppressing the activity of the immune-system cells, which are believed to trigger joint inflammation. It does make sense; some immune-system functions are suppressed naturally during pregnancy so that antibodies in the mother's bloodstream do not perceive the growing fetus as alien to the body and attempt to attack it. It could be that one of those immune-system weapons is the same one that turns renegade and begins to attack the tissues in joints.

## ENDOMETRIOSIS

If you've already had a child, there's little likelihood you'll have to worry about the problem of endometriosis. But it *is* a problem, one from which an estimated 7 percent of all women will suffer. Because it is more common in women who delay childbirth, it's often called "the career woman's disease."

The condition most often strikes a woman between the mid-twenties and forties. Endometriosis is a disease in which the endometrium, the tissue that lines the uterus, grows outside the uterine cavity. When we menstruate, both blood and cells from the endometrium are flushed away. But, in endometriosis, things start to work in reverse: blood and living cells travel backward through the uterus and into the abdominal cavity. What happens next is that these healthy cells attach themselves and begin to grow in places they don't belong: the ovaries, the external surface of the uterus, the fallopian tubes, and even the appendix and bladder.

Once these misplaced cells take hold, they actually respond to hormones as if they were still in the uterus. They begin to multiply in response to the phases of the menstrual cycle. Those of us who experience heavy, long, and frequent periods are more susceptible to endometriosis. Heredity also plays a key role, as the disease tends to run in families.

The most common symptom is agonizing menstrual pain, and in severe cases, the condition can lead to infertility. This in itself is ironic, because one of the surefire cures for endometriosis is to have a child: prolonged resting of the ovaries (anovulation), whether during pregnancy or through drugs, stops the growth of abnormal cells.

A diagnosis of endometriosis can be made much more easily today with the use of a technique called laparoscopy. With the patient under general anesthesia, the surgeon passes a slender tube into the abdomen through a small incision made just below the navel (to minimize the scar). The hollow tube carries a tiny device that lights up the cavity and a telescope-like instrument that allows him to search for telltale signs of the disease in the pelvis or on surrounding tissues. At that time he may destroy small patches of endometriosis tissue by means of an electrical "scalpel" or, more recently, a laser.

The argon laser beam vaporizes the endometriosis tissue and does not harm other organs in the area. It takes about thirty minutes and the patient goes home the same day. So far, no significant side effects have been reported and the pain, sometimes suffered for months, even years, vanishes immediately.

Birth-control pills are often the first line of attack against

155

endometriosis. Because the action of the Pill is to create a hormonal balance similar to that during early pregnancy, the disease can be curtailed, often as well as if the sufferer were actually pregnant. One of the most effective drugs for treating endometriosis is danazol (Danocrine), a synthetic male hormone that blocks ovulation and shrinks the endometrial tissue. However, it also has side effects, which include weight gain and acne.

If a woman has finished her childbearing, the most obvious solution for curing endometriosis is a hysterectomy. But now there is another solution, thanks to laser technology. Traditionally, if severe endometriosis is discovered, the patient is either scheduled for major surgery so the tissue can be removed or is placed on a lengthy course of hormone therapy. Both these methods have serious disadvantages. The surgery requires a large incision in the lower abdomen and often three or four days in the hospital, at a cost of up to $6,000. Hormone therapy usually lasts six to nine months, during which time the woman is unable to conceive, and it can cause such side effects as nausea, vomiting, and excessive fluid retention.

Since the FDA gave the go-ahead for argon lasers to be used, the picture has changed. A main benefit of laser therapy lies in the fact that it can be performed at the time of diagnosis, making it ideal as an outpatient treatment.

The argon laser is a major advance over existing treatments. Not only can it be done on an outpatient basis, but women usually become fertile immediately and at a third of the cost of conventional surgery. William Keye, M.D., chief of the Division of Reproductive Endocrinology and Infertility at the University of Utah School of Medicine, states, "The results have been excellent. It's quick, safe, and much more simple than conventional treatments—with none of the side effects and drawbacks."

Says Dr. Keye: "I have now used argon-laser therapy on almost 300 women and the results have been excellent! Seventy percent of those women for whom endometriosis was the major cause of infertility became pregnant within a year. That figure is better than the results achieved with hormone therapy and about the same as for major surgery. So in terms of cost, safety, and simplicity, the argon-laser treatment is definitely superior." The technique will soon be widely available at medical centers around the country.

# FIBROIDS

One in every four women in our age group—thirty to fifty—will develop tumors in the uterus. Although this may sound alarming, it's really nothing to worry about. Most of these growths are not cancerous.

The most common uterine tumors are fibroids, benign growths made of fibrous and muscular tissue which usually grow in clusters in the muscular layer of the uterus. Among women our age, they are the primary cause of an abnormally enlarged uterus and the number-one reason for hysterectomies. They are often found to run in families: I have known a family in which a mother and her three daughters all needed hysterectomies for fibroids. If the fibroids project into the uterine cavity they will usually cause heavy bleeding at menstruation. If they are large, they can press against other organs: if this happens to the bladder it causes frequent urination; to the intestines it can cause constipation and other changes in bowel movements. Because they are heavy, fibroids can cause chronic backaches and pain from stretched uterine ligaments. The growths can also interfere with conception by preventing a fertilized egg from implanting in the uterus. In pregnant women, fibroids can cause premature labor, miscarriage, and, if very large, difficulty in delivery. Growths that extend from the uterine wall into the pelvic cavity rarely cause any problems and may not even be noticed until discovered during a routine physical. The condition is confirmed with a pelvic ultrasound examination that outlines and measures the tumors.

Because fibroids usually grow slowly, we often just keep them under observation. Obviously, if they grow rapidly we'll think about other options. Keeping an eye on fibroids is particularly important in the case of women approaching menopause. Estrogen stimulates the growth of fibroids, and since estrogen levels decrease after menopause, the tumors often shrink away to nothing. If pregnancy isn't a factor, no other organs are affected, and pain isn't a problem, I much prefer to leave the fibroids alone.

There are, however, some signals that you should pay attention to:

- Heavier than normal periods
- Fatigue (from blood loss)
- Chronic backaches
- Heavy feeling in abdomen, pain and abnormal swelling, or cramps that persist

Hysterectomies now run to about 700,000 operations a year, and half of those are due to fibroids. But now for the good news!

## Myomectomy

There is an alternative surgical technique to a full-blown hysterectomy for coping with fibroids. It's called a myomectomy, the removal of leiomyoma (fibroid). Most surgeons will prefer to perform a hysterectomy: it's quick, relatively simple, and has a good track record for safety. The myomectomy is a little more complicated, but it does have a distinct advantage for women who still want to bear children. The biggest problem surgeons encounter when attempting to remove fibroids is excessive bleeding. In a myomectomy, the surgeon makes an incision through the abdomen and uterus and injects a special solution to retard bleeding. The growths are then re-moved with a scalpel or, in some instances, a laser scalpel. Postoperative recovery from this operation is usually swift, and unlike the radical surgery of a hysterectomy, a myomectomy leaves the patient's reproductive organs intact, so that she is still free to have children.

So, treatment of fibroids depends on your age, whether or not a pregnancy may be desired, and whether or not the growths are either causing you discomfort or making you anemic be-cause of abnormally heavy periods.

## PROBLEMS OF THE CERVIX

You may have been told by your gynecologist that you have a condition called "cervical erosion," and been worried. I've seen patients go into a panic when I tell them this. Actually, it is quite normal, nothing to worry about, and has few or no symptoms.

The term *erosion* is really a misnomer. The condition occurs where the cervix opens into the vagina and two entirely dif-ferent types of cells meet—those of the cervix, which appear rough and shaggy, and those that line the vagina, which are smooth and flat. The cells of the cervix can become more obvious, red and inflamed-looking, as they react to higher estrogen levels—as in the case of the Pill, pregnancy, and during the peak estrogen-producing years. The condition may appear to resemble an erosion, but the correct medical term for it is *eversion* or *ectropion,* meaning simply that the cells may be encroaching into the vaginal area.

However, in our forties and fifties, when ovarian activity and estrogen levels begin to wane, these cells will shrink back into the cervical canal and no longer look or feel "eroded" to the doctor. I'd like to stress a point here: contrary to a popular misconception, the "erosion" cells are definitely not precan-cerous and there is absolutely no need to worry about them.

159

## Cervicitis

This is an acute inflammation of the cervix caused by invading microorganisms. Cervical infections have always been common. With cervicitis, you may notice a vaginal discharge, spotting, pain, and pelvic pressure. The infection may not stay just in the cervix but spread up into the uterus and beyond. This condition can be treated with local or systemic antibiotics, depending on what organism is present.

Both cervicitis and cervical ectropion can result in abnormal Pap-test results. However, I assure you that this in itself is nothing to be alarmed at. In such an event, your physician will simply advise additional tests, such as a repeat Pap after treatment, cervical biopsy, or colposcopy with cervical biopsy.

## Cervical Dysplasia

The cause of this condition is still unknown, but the recent DES controversy has helped to spotlight cervical dysplasia. Many cases of the condition have been discovered in women whose mothers took DES, diethylstilbestrol, a hormone used some fifteen to thirty years ago to treat threatening miscarriages in early pregnancy. Cervical dysplasia has also been found particularly among women who first had sex at an early age and have experienced multiple partners. This gives rise to speculation that the condition may be a sexually transmitted disease with possible connection to the herpes or other viruses. Unfortunately, recent statistics show that women who have had herpes of the genital area or have been infected with the papillomavirus, or HPV, which causes genital warts, are more at risk of developing cancer of the cervix. I tell all my patients who have had herpes or genital warts to be sure, no matter what happens, to have a Pap test every year. I suggest they plan the examination around their birthday because, as years go by, women may get caught up in their careers or families or both and forget to go for an examination—but everyone remembers birthdays!

Technically, the disease is known as cervical intraepithelial neoplasia, or CIN for short. And it's a condition that should not be taken lightly. It is noticeable as an abnormal change in the cells on the wall of the cervix. Here's the big problem: if left untreated, the abnormal development turns into cancer in more than 30 percent of cases. It takes on average about five years for CIN to develop into cervical cancer.

Fortunately, early diagnosis and treatment of CIN can avert the impending disaster of cancer. This is a prime case to illustrate the value of regular Pap tests: in its earliest stages, CIN generally causes no signs or symptoms, but it will be detectable on a simple Pap test! Treatment is relatively easy: cryosurgery, conization, or laser surgery is most often used to destroy the mutant cells before they become cancerous, and in the majority of cases the condition does not reappear. It can be said with optimism that this form of treatment effects a cure if the condition is diagnosed early. Women can rest assured that there is no reason why they should not be able to achieve a successful pregnancy if treatment is begun early enough and has been performed successfully (see cervical cancer, page 197).

# BENIGN BREAST LUMPS

It's one of our worst fears, and especially at this age: discovering a lump in one of our breasts. But let me set you at ease. Despite universal anxiety, the vast majority of breast lumps are in no way cancerous. Now, this doesn't mean it's time to take breast lumps less seriously; it just means that you don't have to panic if you do discover one. There are five different types of breast lumps that are essentially harmless and nothing to worry about.

Benign lumps occur in the breast tissue of 50 percent of women: they will usually be one of the following five types:

*Intraductal papilloma.* This is a small, harmless growth inside a milk duct, just beneath the nipple. Surgery is usually

161

recommended for the removal of these lumps. A tiny incision around the nipple is possible so that the breast is not deformed.

*Fibrocystic disease.* These lumps affect 1 in 3 women at some time in their life, usually appearing just before the menstrual period and diminishing rapidly afterward. Made up of several small lumps, the condition makes your breast feel like a cobbled street. The lumps are thought to be caused by fluctuations in the levels of estrogen. A number of studies have shown that reducing consumption of caffeine and high-fat foods—particularly red meat and cheese—can reduce them.

*Fibroadenomas.* Solid, round, smooth, and freely movable, this benign tumor feels like a marble just under the skin. The lumps are rarely cancerous but should be removed for definitive diagnosis. It's a simple procedure, usually under local anesthesia.

*Cysts.* These firm, fluid-filled sacs may appear suddenly and are frequently painful. If they do not subside after menstruation you should have a mammogram to make sure that the swelling is indeed a cyst; it can often be treated by drawing off the fluid with a needle.

*Hematoma.* This is caused by an injury. A lump appears beneath the bruised area and may be painful or tender for days or weeks. Like any bump from an injury, it should slowly disappear as the blood clot below the skin's surface is absorbed. If not, the lump may require a tiny incision to drain the fluid.

But remember, *any* lump should be examined by your doctor for your own peace of mind.


## ULCERS

Here's an area in which we females have made great strides—unfortunately, they're in the wrong direction! Fifty years ago, only about one in twenty ulcer cases involved women; today it's one in two. Over the years, I've noticed a definite increase in the number of wives and mothers who come to me complaining of pain that turns out to be due to stomach (gastric) or duodenal ulcers. Now the trend is more toward the career woman.

Ulcers should be of particular concern to women our age. Many may be returning to the work force for the first time after raising families. Others of the more valiant among us may be juggling two life-styles, raising kids and holding down a full-time job. And then there are our professional career women, now hitting their prime and possibly feeling increased pressures of climbing the corporate ladder.

Stress has been known for years to be a major precipitating factor in ulcer disease. Patients will demonstrate recurrence of symptoms at times of increased stress and healing takes place as stress levels fall. Ulcer patients are often chronically anxious and have a negative outlook on life. Stress increases the flow of gastric acids in the stomach, as do coffee (even the decaffeinated kind) and other caffeinated beverages and alcohol (including beer). An additional hazard is cigarette smoking: smokers have twice the incidence of ulcers than nonsmokers and the risk of gastric ulcer correlates with the number of cigarettes smoked. Aspirin and other nonsteroidal anti-inflammatory drugs (NSAIDs) also damage the epithelial lining of the stomach, as do steroid drugs (e.g., cortisone) occasionally. I have always found a family history to be present in women who have ulcers: they tell me their father or mother or sibling also had ulcer disease.

So maybe it's really no surprise that more of us are experiencing the agonies of ulcers in this day and age. Certainly women are drinking more alcohol and smoking more cigarettes than ever before. Those of you who continually take aspirin, especially for stress-induced headaches, should be aware of these facts.

Ulcers, by the way, are not what many people imagine. They are not eruptions in the stomach or duodenum—the section of the small intestine that attaches to the lower portion of the stomach—but rather raw patches of exposed tissue. A peptic

ulcer resembles a crater in the lining of the stomach or duodenum. It is formed when gastric juices, for some still not
quite understood reason, eat away a small portion of the digestive tract. Under normal circumstances, the walls of our digestive organs are well equipped to withstand the powerful acids
and highly caustic enzymes, like pepsin, that break down and
digest our foods. The protection comes from a layer of mucus
that coats the membrane that lines the stomach and duodenum. But sometimes either the protective mucus breaks
down and/or we begin to produce increased amounts of digestive fluids.

Although peptic ulcers can occur in the stomach, they are
ten times more likely to erupt in the duodenum.

## Myths Abound

Once it was accepted that the only way to treat an ulcer was
to stick rigidly to a bland diet. And, once upon a time, milk
was prescribed as the staple drink for ulcer sufferers. Now it
is known that after its calmative effect, milk can actually ex-
acerbate the problem by producing an increase in stomach
acid. Loading the stomach with antacids and chalky calcium
drinks and tablets was another way to combat ulcers, but research has shown that that can cause problems as well, most
notably with the kidneys.

## The Latest Treatments

The best way to attack ulcers is by reducing the output of
gastric secretions. It seems logical and cost-effective to try first
a regime of a caffeine- and alcohol-free diet, avoiding irritant
drugs and trying seriously to reduce stress. If this does not
work, today's treatment of choice is a drug called Tagamet
(cimetidine) which works like magic to reduce gastric acid, thus
allowing the body to heal the ulcerated mucosa.[2]

And would you believe it, here comes pregnancy to the

rescue again! Studies have shown that women who get pregnant almost always find that their ulcer symptoms disappear. What's the secret? It looks like it's estrogen, this time as a seemingly natural ally against ulcers. Although I am not aware of any studies that have performed clinical trials on ulcer sufferers, it might be sensible to theorize that the estrogen boosts we get from the Pill may also play a role in reducing the incidence of ulcers.

The bottom line on ulcers is to seek immediate treatment. Apart from the obvious pain and discomfort they cause, ulcers can lead to dangerous complications.

# VAGINITIS

About half of all complaints heard by a gynecologist are descriptions of symptoms of vaginitis. The condition is an inflammation or infection of the vaginal canal and can be caused by fungus or bacteria. The telltale signs are burning and itching and an abnormal discharge that can vary in color, odor, and texture. In fact, vaginitis is so common that most of us women will suffer from it at one time in our lives.

Whether you realize it or not, the vagina is alive with a whole host of organisms that usually cause no harm and actually act to prevent against infections. They help maintain the proper acid-alkaline balance of the vagina, which is normally slightly acidic. If that balance changes more to the alkaline, it provides an ideal breeding ground for numerous opportunistic organisms. Because blood itself is alkaline, the pH in the vagina rises during menstruation, making you particularly susceptible to infection during your periods.

The most common causes of vaginitis are:

***Candida albicans,*** a yeastlike fungus that results in a thick white discharge looking something like cottage cheese and smelling like baked bread. Those of us who are pregnant, diabetic, run-down, or using birth-control pills—all conditions that change the normal pH of the vagina—are most at risk from yeast infections. Candida (known more commonly as *monilia*) can be a problem after a woman takes certain antibiotics for any kind of infection. The antibiotics kill off the "good-guy" bacteria in the vagina as well as the tonsillitis or bronchitis germs for which they were originally meant. Now the monilia can grow unrestrained, causing severe itching and irritation. If you know you are susceptible to this problem, tell your doctor when he prescribes medication for an infection, so that he can give you something to counter the expected upsurge of monilia. Yeast infections are easily treated by antifungal creams or vaginal suppositories. I occasionally recommend douching with plain yogurt, which contains bacteria that are natural enemies of yeast.

*Trichomonas vaginalis,* or "trich," is a one-celled protozoan that causes approximately 2.5 million cases of infection among us annually, with one out of five women suffering from it during their sexually active years. It is usually recognizable by a frothy, thin, yellow-greenish discharge that has an offensive odor. Symptoms include intense itching, redness, and frequent, painful urination. Although most often transmitted through sexual contact, trich can be picked up from wet towels, bathing suits, or underwear. The most effective treatment for this condition is a drug called metronidazole (Flagyl). Other treatments include Betadine gels and douches and a new cream called Vagetrol.

*Hemophilus vaginalis* is a bacterium that causes a greyish, gelatinous discharge that sometimes has an odor. Burning and itching are the signs to look for. Sulfonamide creams are effective in mild cases, but stronger antibiotics may be necessary in stubborn cases.

A few tips to help prevent vaginitis: don't eat too much sugar, as it tends to affect the vagina's normal pH; always wipe yourself from front to back so there's less chance of bacteria spreading from the rectum to the vaginal entrance; keep the area of the vulva clean and dry; and whenever possible, wear cotton or cotton-paneled underwear, which will not trap moisture and heat—ideal breeding conditions for unwanted organisms.

# VENEREAL DISEASE

## Chlamydia

The "new" lovebug is an organism called chlamydia. The disease is a very old one, known from ancient times. But the ability to detect the organism is a very recent and welcome development. Today it's the nation's number-one sexually transmitted disease and strikes nearly 10 million women every year.

Often described as the "silent disease" because initially it's virtually symptomless, chlamydia is taking a devastating toll. Left untreated, it's a cause of 50 percent of cases of potentially serious pelvic inflammatory disease (PID), and therefore a major cause of tubal pregnancy and infertility. Chlamydia responds well to drugs, but, unfortunately, most women are unaware they're infected, so treatment often begins only when serious complications develop.

Until recently, there has not been a quick, inexpensive, and readily available way of screening women for chlamydia infections. The traditional test—by which all others are compared—is a tissue culture. This involves gently removing material from the lining of the cervix with a swab and then analyzing it in the laboratory. Such cultures are expensive, however—as much as $80—and few labs are equipped to do them.

However, a new blood test is now showing promising results. Called an antigen detection test (ADT), it provides answers in thirty minutes—compared with three to five days with tissue cultures—and costs around $20. Preliminary results suggest that the test accurately detects chlamydia infections even in

167

patients who have no symptoms. It could become an excellent screening technique.

I routinely offer any woman who is sexually active a test for chlamydia which has been available for about two years. A swab is taken from the cervix or the urethra to collect cells, which are carefully smeared on a slide. When the slide is stained with a fluorescent dye, the electron microscope easily picks up this intracellular organism which shows on the slide as a bright green dot inside the cells. The test costs about $18 and is 92 percent accurate. I strongly recommend that women have this test done: if you keep with the same faithful partner, it does not have to be repeated.

Occasionally, I've seen women develop early symptoms: painful urination, painful intercourse, a thick, creamy genital discharge. The cervix may also become swollen and reddened and there may be bleeding. Such symptoms usually appear within seven to fourteen days of being exposed to the organism. Even though symptoms may vanish without treatment, the infection remains and can be passed on to others. The partner of a positive case must be treated. Women may be infected, have no symptoms, and the infection may be silent for years.

Because as many as 13 percent of pregnant women have the bacteria in the cervix, and 70 percent of babies born to these women will be infected, some doctors are recommending that all pregnant women should have a chlamydia test.

Tetracycline antibiotics—like doxycycline—are the most effective form of treatment. Pregnant women are usually given erythromycin. With the disease so rampant, it is important that all sexually active women see their gynecologist for chlamydia testing, not only to avoid serious complications, but also to enjoy peace of mind.

## Gonorrhea

This disease may affect as many as 2 million women every year. And it's a major health threat because it can lead to pelvic inflammatory disease. It's caused by the gonococcus bacterium and is spread by sexual contact; but many women may not initially realize they have contracted the disease, owing to the lack of early symptoms. When symptoms finally do arrive, they often include painful urination and intercourse, vaginal discharge, unusual vaginal bleeding, pelvic pain, tenderness, and even fever.

If the infection isn't treated early, it can spread through the reproductive tract to your uterus and fallopian tubes, where it can cause serious damage. At that stage the symptoms are usually severe abdominal pain, muscle aches, nausea, fever, and chills. Infertility, repeated hard-to-control infections, and persistent pain are usually the long-term result.

If you think you have an infection go and be tested: it could be gonorrhea, which is serious but is usually easy to treat. Injections of penicillin almost always cure the condition before it can reach an advanced stage. If you do become infected, avoid any sex until you have been treated, and try to make sure that your partner does the same. Using a condom does afford some protection, both from catching the disease and from spreading it.

## Pelvic Inflammatory Disease (PID)

Pelvic inflammatory disease can occur in any woman at any age. At least 85,000 women every year suffer from the condition, the results of which are annually increasing rates of tubal pregnancy and infertility.

Your biggest enemies when it comes to PID are chlamydia and gonorrhea. A woman's reproductive tract has wonderful defenses against microorganisms, but these two leading causes of VD are very virulent and certainly on the increase, especially chlamydia. The infecting organisms travel up through the cervix and the uterus to the fallopian tubes which become inflamed, hot, and tender to the examiner's touch or during intercourse. The ovary may also be involved: the disease may be on one side of the pelvis or on both sides. Abscesses may form, and scar tissue which may obstruct the tubes. Adhesions can develop between the tubes and ovaries and the adjacent bowel or bladder, making infertility likely. The condition may be indolent, with few symptoms, or cause pain of different degrees, occasionally very severe on any kind of movement. There is often discharge and fever: a blood count shows evidence of infection. Mild cases can be treated with oral antibiotics and rest; however, if the condition is allowed to persist, other bacteria can crowd in to worsen it, and a hospital stay with intravenous antibiotics may be necessary. In the worst of cases, surgery may have to be performed to remove scar tissue or even the entire uterus, tubes, and ovaries.

Prevention is absolutely the best bet when dealing with PID, and that means early recognition and treatment of venereal diseases such as chlamydia and gonorrhea.

## THE HONEYMOON DISEASE

Many of us may first notice it during or after a prolonged surge of sexual activity—hence the name "honeymoon cystitis." More than half of us will develop a bladder infection at some time in our lives.

Interestingly, the woman in her fifth decade may be more prone to encountering this problem, for a couple of reasons: first, she may, possibly because of divorce or the pressure of the family-raising years, have been refraining from heavy sexual activity and may now be experiencing a sexual reawakening; second, the tissues of the vagina and urethra are thinning because of estrogen depletion and are much less resistant to infection.

The problem is urinary tract infection (UTI), which most often occurs when bacteria that normally live in the intestine find their way into the bladder or urethra. When they invade the urethra, the infection is called urethritis; when the bladder, cystitis. Both, if left untreated, can lead to more serious prob-

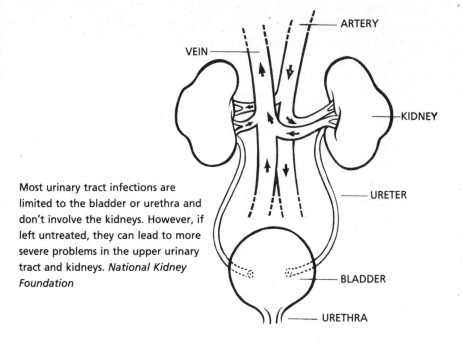

Most urinary tract infections are limited to the bladder or urethra and don't involve the kidneys. However, if left untreated, they can lead to more severe problems in the upper urinary tract and kidneys. *National Kidney Foundation*

## THE KIDNEYS AND KIDNEY INFECTION

lems in the upper urinary tract and the kidneys. Suspect kidney infection if you have chills, backache, fever, or vomiting.

Common symptoms of lower tract UTI are: painful urination caused by urine passing through the inflamed neck of the bladder; urgency and pain after voiding; frequent nighttime urination; pain and cramping in the lower abdomen; and cloudy and sometimes bloody urine. We are more prone to urinary infections than men because the space between the rectum and the vagina is small, making it easier for bacteria to migrate into the vagina. Our urethras are also shorter than the male version, so the invading organisms have less distance to travel before multiplying and starting up an infection.

You may be surprised to know that there are some contributing factors to cystitis that are easily overlooked. Poor hygiene is the most obvious, but vaginal creams, possibly the use of a diaphragm, and even some "hygiene" sprays and douches can lead to UTI. Because chilling the lower body can predispose a woman to cystitis, I tell women of all ages not to sit around in a damp bathing suit.

There are other measures you can follow to help in prevention. The best protection against UTI is to drink lots of fluids and empty the bladder at regular intervals. Responding to the urge to urinate helps flush bacteria out of the urinary tract. I can also recommend drinking lots of cranberry juice at the first hint of a cystitis problem. No, it's not an old wives' tale. Cranberry juice (but not citrus juices) is high in acidity and increases the acidity of the urine, making it a more inhospitable environment for unwanted bacteria. Alcohol, tea, coffee, and spicy foods are to be avoided because they can further inflame the bladder.

Treatment of a UTI is with an appropriate antibiotic which kills all the bacteria in the bladder and urethra, usually a sulfonamide. If you are having a lot of burning or pain you may be given a drug to relieve those symptoms and it is always necessary to drink large quantities of fluids, up to a gallon a day. This keeps the urine dilute and flushes out the kidneys and bladder. A one-day large single-shot dose of antibiotic may be tried for mild cases of UTI, usually after the urine is tested under the microscope for white blood cells and set up for culture in the laboratory. Severe cases should have antibiotics for ten to fourteen days and when the infection is in the kidneys treatment may have to be for four to eight weeks and hospitalization may be necessary.

Some women have frequent episodes of cystitis or urethritis related to sexual activity. Prevention tactics include drinking lots of extra fluids before intercourse and emptying your bladder immediately afterward. Your doctor may prescribe an active antibiotic to take just after sexual contact that will prevent reinfection. If you do have symptoms of UTI at any time, take active measures immediately so as to prevent the infection from finding its way to your kidneys.

*Note for pregnant women:* Some 10 percent of pregnant women will develop a UTI. Although this number may seem small, as the problem leads to an increased chance of miscarriage or premature labor, it's a good idea for any pregnant woman to be monitored on a regular basis for UTIs, even if she has no symptoms.

## RECURRENT UTIs

It is a good idea if a woman has two or more attacks of cystitis or one severe kidney infection to have an ultrasound or X-ray examination of the kidneys, intravenous pyelogram (IVP). I tell my patients that it is important to identify any obstruction in the urinary tract from the kidneys to the ureters to the bladder and urethra. Ultrasound is advantageous because it does not involve radiation and will show up many abnormalities of the kidneys or ureters: sometimes an IVP is necessary to outline the inner parts of the kidney and to see if the urine flows back up the ureter from the bladder (ureteral reflux). It is crucial to treat any condition causing interference with free flow of the urine as the kidneys can be damaged by repeated infections. Many of these conditions are easily corrected with modern surgical techniques.

## WARTS

Genital warts are now the third most common sexually transmitted disease in the United States. A million men and women seek medical care for this human papilloma virus infection each year—about three times as many as are treated for genital herpes. And with the growing number of single women in their forties, this is a problem many of us should be concerned about.

A woman without symptoms may learn of the infection in one of three ways: from her partner, from her gynecologist at the time of a routine examination, or from the results of a Pap smear.

Genital warts, or condylomata accuminata, appear as painless, fleshy growths, usually no larger than the tip of a pencil, occurring singly or in clusters. They often cause itching, burning, or mild discomfort in the genital area, especially the perineal area (the region between vagina and anus).

Like many forms of venereal disease, genital warts can be transmitted unknowingly by people who have few or no symptoms. In the person exposed to someone with this condition, it may take two or three months or more for the warts to appear. During the latency period, the virus may be present, spreading during sexual activity. It is customary to do a blood test for syphilis, a VDRL, as this disease may also cause venereal warts which, although not identical, must be differentiated from condylomata accuminata.

Treatment can be frustrating because these warts tend to recur; the virus often remains in the body even after they have been removed. Application of a solution called podophyllin provides effective relief for most cases of external warts. Those inside the vagina or on the cervix respond to trichloracetic acid (TCA). Genital warts can also be removed by freezing, an outpatient procedure called cryosurgery. And laser surgery is the latest weapon being aimed at these annoying growths.

One of the most important steps in stopping the spread of venereal warts is the use of condoms. Warts are highly infectious, transmitted only by sexual intercourse; the chance of getting them from an infected partner is greater than 50 percent. So, if you're single and sexually active, insist that your partner use a condom.

Women need to know that having had infection with human papilloma virus makes them at increased risk for developing cervical cancer. So annual Pap tests are a must for those who have had this condition.

# KIDNEY STONES

While we're still on the subject of our waterworks and internal plumbing, it's opportune to raise the question of kidney stones (renal calculi). You are at the age when kidney stones are most likely to appear simply because in most cases they take many years to form.

Kidney stones are still a medical mystery. In about 80 percent of cases, there is no indication of what caused them to form in the first place, although we know that there is a strong connection between kidney stones and heredity. The good news for us women is that we tend to form "silent," or painless, stones, while men are more likely to develop stones that cause agonizing pain. The many different causes of stone formation will be investigated by your doctor through blood tests and most importantly by analysis of the stone itself. It is extremely important to catch the stone as it passes out in the urine so it can be chemically studied. If you suspect renal colic, when you pass your urine, strain it through coffee-filter paper or gauze.

When it strikes, the pain of kidney stones has been described as one of the most excruciating experiences known to humankind. The pain can hit right out of the blue, striking with debilitating swiftness. It can be so intense that the sufferer will keel over and faint or break out into a sweat. The pain usually strikes in the flank on the side of the affected kidney. It can be felt in the back and can radiate right down into the groin or bladder area. The urge to urinate is usually present at the same time. The pain comes and goes in waves and will move down the body as the stone moves down the urinary tract.

Most kidney stones are small, measuring no more than a couple of millimeters in diameter, and will be passed naturally out of the body in a matter of a few hours or days. Larger stones may take days and even weeks, and these may be cause for medical intervention. So if you know you have a small stone or "gravel," you will hope to be able to pass it by drinking lots of liquids and using medication for pain.

More good news: the two latest innovations in the treatment of kidney stones may make surgical removal obsolete. One is to effectively destroy the stones by breaking them up with sound waves (lithotripsy).[3] The sufferer is immersed in a bath of water and the kidney is bombarded with focused ultrasound. The shock waves, while not affecting tissue, will reduce the stones to fine sand, or at least much smaller fragments, which can then eventually pass out of the body. Percutaneous nephrostomy, the second new technique, involves passing a tiny catheter through the body and into the affected kidney. Ultrasonic lithotripsy to shatter stones or chemicals that are able to dissolve them are then carefully fed through the catheter directly to the site of the offending calculi.

Once you've had a stone in the urinary tract, you must remember to keep your urine dilute at all times, especially in hot weather, by drinking lots of fluids. This may prevent reoccurrence.

## KEEPING CONTROL

A common physical change a woman may notice in her forties is a tendency to leak a few drops of urine. Don't be upset or fearful about this: it is usually nothing to worry about.

Bladder incontinence, often known as stress incontinence, is a product of aging. It most often affects women who have had several children and is a consequence of the stresses and strains placed upon the female design. The two main causes are a decrease in estrogen levels and the stretching of the pelvic floor muscles and other tissues that support the bladder. It is

Although a fair amount is known about the circumstances and consequences of stone formation, the mechanisms still remain obscure. For instance, urine normally contains chemical substances that inhibit the formation of crystals, but no one knows why these inhibitors do not work for everyone. *National Kidney Foundation*

RENAL PELVIS

STONE

URETER

STONE

BLADDER

STONE

BLADDER NECK

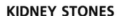

**KIDNEY STONES**

not unusual, especially if the bladder is full, to leak a little urine when you laugh, sneeze, or cough.

However, incontinence may indicate an underlying disorder of a more serious nature. Certain neurological disease states can cause incontinence, as can urinary tract infections that need immediate treatment.

For the vast majority of cases of incontinence, the amount of urine that leaks is so minimal that wearing a small sanitary pad during times of physical stress may be all that is necessary to avoid any embarrassment. Most of the women I see with this problem come to me when the condition has become socially unacceptable, when they can no longer go to exercise classes and keep dry, or when an irritation develops from constantly wearing a pad.

Fortunately, there are some easy steps you can take to improve the situation. The most widely prescribed approach is the Kegel exercises, which build up pelvic muscle tone (see page 95).

In many cases, surgery may be necessary and is nearly always successful. A wonderful new technique is now showing a lot of promise. The procedure involves inserting thin metal supports along the pelvic floor to give it added support. Latest results show a better than 95 percent success rate with quick recovery and few complications. Most women wish they had considered the surgery earlier to relieve these uncomfortable symptoms.


## THAT OTHER ITCH!

Hemorrhoids—the problem none of us likes to discuss. We've blamed just about everything for the cause of this embarrassing condition, from the strain of walking on two legs to the comforts of indoor plumbing, which allow us to sit instead of squat to perform our most natural of functions.

Like it or not, hemorrhoids are common and we are in the age range when they are most likely to start acting up, if they haven't already. Very similar to varicose veins, they are blood vessels around the anus and rectum that become weakened and stretched. The cause is believed to be an inherited weakness in the vessel walls themselves. And it may be small comfort, but if you suffer from this itching and often painful problem, you are not alone; there are millions more women suffering right along with you.

Hemorrhoids often develop during pregnancy because of

increased pressure on pelvic veins and after delivery because the pressure of the baby's head stretches out the blood vessels around the anus. Chronic constipation, and the stress and strain of coping with it, has the same effect.

Internal hemorrhoids develop inside the rectum, cause bleeding problems, and occasionally need surgical treatment. Those around the opening of the rectum or that protrude outside the anus are known as external hemorrhoids. Because they are more abundant in sensitive nerves, they frequently cause intense itching, burning, and pain.

Home care of hemorrhoids is most often as near as your bathtub. The moist heat from bathing is effective in reducing inflammation. Some medications available over the counter are helpful, but in more severe cases your physician can prescribe suppositories or ointments.

The best bet for hemorrhoids is to try and avoid them altogether. Eating a lot of fiber and exercising regularly are the safest ways to beat the strain of constipation. Taking laxatives is not a good idea because they can cause diarrhea, which in turn may further irritate the already inflamed vessels.

Surgical removal of hemorrhoids is strongly recommended for women who have ongoing problems of bleeding or pain. The relief is enormous, and I find that most women will say after surgery, "I should have had that done years ago!"

# FEMININE HYGIENE

A word on another sensitive subject—douching. It's a controversial subject today. For centuries, women have tried it to relieve almost every kind of vaginal disorder. To hear the advertisements for douching products, you'd think they were an absolute necessity for feminine hygiene.

Though there is little scientific data concerning the risks and benefits of douching, most physicians feel that it has little medical value. If practiced occasionally and sensibly, douching is rarely harmful. But doing it excessively or using harsh ingredients can be hazardous.

The vagina is a self-cleaning organ. Normal secretions of mucus wash out foreign matter and protect the vaginal walls. In addition, a healthy woman harbors many different types of microorganisms in her vagina, including bacteria that fight infection. While one mild douche is unlikely to upset this delicate balance, frequent douching can strip away protective mucus and kill helpful bacteria.

There have been numerous cases of women suffering chemical peritonitis—a dangerous inflammation of the abdominal lining—from forcing the douche solution through the uterus and into the abdominal cavity by using too much pressure.

If you have a vaginal infection—they're common at our age—douching will wash away the thick discharge that burns or itches but the relief is temporary. The infection will not be cured, and the itch will return. Only your doctor's prescription can cure the infection.

It is particularly important not to douche before a gynecological examination for vaginitis. Your doctor needs to examine the discharge to make the correct diagnosis.

While an infection can produce an unpleasant smell, normal vaginal odor, if present at all, is slight and inoffensive. Advertising may have convinced the public otherwise, but you should be aware that the perfumes and deodorants in some douche products can irritate the vagina.

Still, studies show that at least 60 percent of women douche occasionally. If you feel better about yourself by douching, by all means do so—but not too often; that means once a month at most. And I tell my patients there is really no reason they should find it necessary at all.

## The Talc Dilemma

Talcum powder is one of the most widely used of all bath products. You can also find it in an assortment of products from eyeliners to rouge, foot powders to deodorants. It may look inoffensive, but a debate is now stirring over talc's safety. There is now a great deal of circumstantial evidence showing that talc can cause ovarian cancer.

Many women use it on a daily basis to dust the area around the vagina and the anus. Studies have shown that particles of powder containing talcum find their way into the vagina and turn up in the fallopian tubes as soon as thirty minutes later. From here the talc makes its way to the ovaries, where it can trigger changes that cause cancer. But, I repeat: this is *circumstantial* evidence; no definitive link has been proved between the use of such powders and the development of ovarian cancer. Nevertheless, as the *possibility* of a link does exist, I advise my patients not to use talcum powder but that, if they wish, cornstarch (used in baby powder) is safe.

As women, we do face a myriad of potential problems, some—like the ones described above—less serious than others. Next we are going to tackle the major ones.

# 7

# Major Concerns

Of all the health concerns we face today, cancer and heart disease are the biggest killers of women. But it doesn't have to be this way. For decades, women in general have relied too much on scant medical supervision and not enough on their own feelings, instincts, and educated intuition to recognize when their bodies are at risk and possibly developing problems. Nipping in the bud diseases like cancer and heart disease is the most positive route to effect an eventual cure. When these diseases are caught early, they are highly treatable, often without hospitalization; when left to develop, they may result in horrendous medical bills, family anguish, and ultimately death.

With the superior screening methods available today—especially the latest mammography techniques for breast cancer, Pap tests, and more sophisticated methods for early detection of cervical cancer—it is hoped that women will stop dying from these conditions. Of course, it is your initial awareness that can save the day, and the more information you have at your fingertips, the easier it is to spot these potentially life-threatening diseases.

In my own practice I am very much aware of the value of breast self-examination. You are much more likely to find a lump early if you are in the habit of checking yourself regularly. It is estimated that as many as 80 percent of women discover their own cancerous lesion first. It has been shown that physical examination by a physician and screening mammography diagnose cancer at an earlier stage and are crucial ways to combat this life-threatening disease. So, learn to examine your breasts and work with your physician as partners to try to prevent breast cancer. (See also page 200.)

# HEART DISEASE

One of the wonders of our female body is that we have a built-in, mysterious protective shield against heart disease. While our fifth-decade male friends have been running around for the past few years facing a distinct risk of heart disease, we have been blithely floating along without a care in the world. I hate to be a killjoy, but our cardiac protection is coming to an end. The closer we come to menopause, the more shaky that protective shield becomes.

The reason I refer to this protective factor we enjoy as a "mystery" is that we haven't quite pinned down yet what it is. It was once believed that high levels of estrogen were responsible, but in studies of men who were given doses of estrogen, their incidence of heart attack actually increased. It is most likely that the secret does lie in estrogen, although it might be a combination of estrogen with other female hormones and that effect may be unique to women.

Coronary artery disease, or atherosclerosis, while extremely rare among women in their 30s, accounts for approximately 60 deaths per 100,000 in the female population, and overall it is still by far the biggest killer we face. The annual incidence rate of the disease is 31 per 10,000 among women ages 45 to 54, after which it increases threefold to 95 per 10,000 between ages 55 and 64. Diseases of the heart and blood vessels kill

1,200,000 Americans each year, and that's about 2½ times as many as are killed by cancer, 9 times as many as will succumb to accidental death, and almost 17 times as many as those who will perish from pneumonia or influenza.

As we enter our 40s, our chances of heart attack are believed to lag about 8 years behind those of men. In other words, a woman of 45 may be considered to face the same risks as a man of 37. But, unfortunately for us, there's a catch here: if we do experience cardiac problems, they are much more likely to be of a serious nature than are those experienced by our male counterparts. Consider this: of women who suffer a heart attack, 45 percent die within the first year, compared with a figure of only 20 percent for males. During the first five years, the comparison is even worse: the recurrence rate for women is around 40 percent, while it's not much over 10 percent for men. I'm often asked why this should be so, and the honest answer is that neither I nor anybody else in the medical profession knows.

## What Is a Heart Attack?

In simple terms, it is the end product of the effect of a portion of the heart muscle being starved of its vital blood supply. For the heart to continue to be healthy, it needs its own nourishing supply of blood, which is provided through the coronary vessels. Contrary to what many people think, a heart attack is not the heart losing its ability to pump, but something that is intervening to block the heart's own lifeline, its supply of blood. Heart attacks have many faces. In fact, no two heart attacks are ever exactly the same, because of the varying degrees of damage inflicted on the heart muscle, the myocardium, and location of the myocardial damage when the electrical mechanism of the heart may be affected, causing abnormal rhythms which may be fatal. While the symptoms of attack may also differ, the end product—the survivability factor—is gauged by the location and how much tissue and how many cells in that particular area of the heart have survived.

No heart attack is ever considered as a minor event, but some of you may already have had one and never even known it. The fleeting pain in the chest was probably passed off as a muscle spasm or indigestion. This is said not to alarm you, only to alert you. Obviously the transient attack didn't do enough damage to the myocardium to alter the heart's functioning. Consequently it went unnoticed. Even so, a trained physician may pick up a telltale clue on an electrocardiogram at a later date. Don't be lulled into a false sense of security here, as the

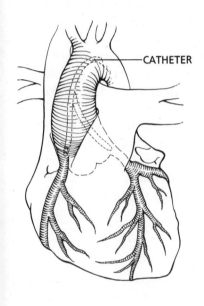

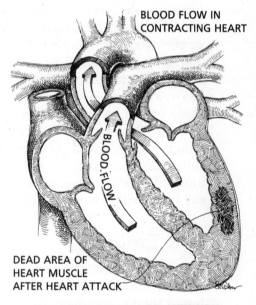

## CORONARY ARTERIOGRAPHY

This diagram displays how a catheter can be threaded through major arteries into the heart. A dye is then pumped into the coronary vessels to pinpoint potential problems. *American Heart Association*

## EFFECTS OF HEART ATTACK

The result of a nonfatal heart attack. Note the area of dead heart muscle—the result of oxygen starvation caused by inadequate blood supply. *American Heart Association*

185

existence of a previous attack, no matter how minor, is a sure indicator that problems are in store and that coronary disease is beginning to build up. The massive coronary occlusion, of course, is the one we must be deeply concerned about. Coronary arteries become narrowed by the buildup of fatty deposits, or atheromatous plaque, on the inside walls of the vessel. When the artery becomes totally blocked, the area of heart muscle it supplies loses its blood supply (becomes ischemic), and therefore the necessary oxygen for its functioning (becomes hypoxic). If this ischemia lasts long enough the cells in the heart muscle die from lack of oxygen: the end result is tissue death (necrosis) which is called an infarction. A myocardial infarction, MI, is thus caused by a coronary occlusion or coronary thrombosis (a blood clot in the coronary artery). The severity of an MI or heart attack clearly depends on how much of the myocardium is damaged. Remember the heart has to keep beating at least 50 times every minute through all these events. What is amazing is that a small infarction will heal and the surrounding heart muscle will be oxygenated by blood diverted from other nearby vessels, a safeguard called collateral circulation. If the myocardial damage is extensive and collateral vessels cannot supply adequate circulation, then the heart will fail and death will ensue.

## Risk Factors

With more and more women working today, we doctors have feared an increase in female heart-attack rates. According to the Framingham Heart Study—an ongoing years-long project that is following entire generations of the populace of Framingham, Massachusetts—there is no overall statistical difference in the incidence of heart disease between women who worked outside the home and those who are housewives. However, one subgroup, those women with clerical and sales jobs, approaches the same rate of heart disease as men. Working women with children also appear to have a higher risk of heart

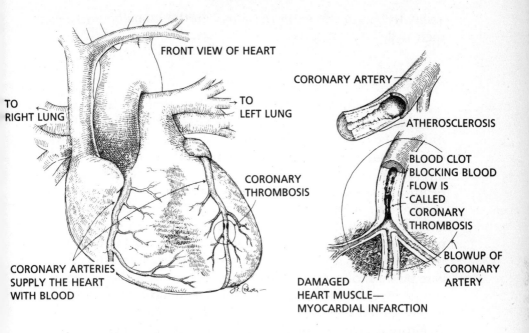

FRONT VIEW OF HEART

CORONARY ARTERY

TO
RIGHT LUNG

TO
LEFT LUNG

ATHEROSCLEROSIS

CORONARY
THROMBOSIS

BLOOD CLOT
BLOCKING BLOOD
FLOW IS
CALLED
CORONARY
THROMBOSIS

CORONARY ARTERIES
SUPPLY THE HEART
WITH BLOOD

BLOWUP OF
CORONARY
ARTERY

DAMAGED
HEART MUSCLE—
MYOCARDIAL INFARCTION

## CORONARY THROMBOSIS (effects of blood clot)

These drawings illustrate how the cardiac vessels supply the heart with blood
and the result of atherosclerosis which can lead to potentially fatal blood
clots and heart attack. *American Heart Association*

disease than those without kids. The highest incidence of heart
problems—even higher than the average incidence among
males—is found in a small group of female clerical workers
who have children. This phenomenon is believed to be linked
to the stress/heart disease connection; people who have high-
stress life-styles traditionally are more at risk for coronary
disease. On the whole, the lower incidence of heart problems
among the general population of women can best be explained
by two factors: the not yet fully understood protection af-
forded by the younger female body, and women's apparent

ability to handle stress on the job or in the home better than their male counterparts.

## Stress

It is well known that stress plays a major part in the drama of a heart attack. This may mean stress on the job with a difficult boss or coworkers, ongoing tensions in a business venture that is not going well, or day-to-day fast-lane living in a very competitive world. Stress at home may be acute (illness, death, or separation and divorce) or chronic (an unhappy marriage or living with an emotionally unbalanced partner, children, or parents). Some people handle stress better than others: the term "Type A behavior" has been used to describe the behavior of people who are prone to coronary artery disease because of a personality characterized by a short fuse, a competitive, hostile attitude to others, and a constant sense of urgency. In a new book,[1] Dr. David L. Copen and Dr. Mark Rubinstein give excellent examples of typical stresses in patients' lives and follow with suggestions of ways to combat stress in a major effort to prevent coronary thrombosis in susceptible individuals.

Although most people think of the Type A person as a male, we all know that women also fit this description. As women take on more positions of responsibility in the business and professional world, they should know how to reduce stress to protect their hearts.

## The Pill

We've heard mostly good news about the Pill, but here's the negative side. The risk of heart attack attributed to oral contraceptives used by women of forty and over is more than twelve times that of females in their thirties. Among younger women, the heart-problem risk is not considered a serious threat, certainly not enough to warrant their coming off the

Pill unless other risk factors are involved. The risk factor increases greatly for women if they are both on the Pill and are also smokers.

## Obesity

Being overweight places a tremendous strain on the heart. Men and women have somewhat different weight-gain profiles. Both sexes gain weight—if they're going to—mostly between the ages of eighteen and fifty. However, men tend to stay the same weight once they reach fifty, whereas women tend to continue gaining into their fifties and even sixties. Obesity is clearly linked with the development of hypertension which is a risk factor for coronary artery disease and other forms of heart disease. The message for those of us in our forties, therefore, is to try and establish a leaner profile during this decade to offset the weight-gaining years to come.

I believe an easy rule of thumb to follow for good health is to stick to a weight that is no more than 10 percent over the "ideal" weight range for your height and body frame (see weight tables in Chapter 2). Anything over 20 percent of the norm starts to run into the unhealthy category.

## High Blood Pressure

It's called "the silent killer," and for good reason. Increasingly more cardiologists are citing high blood pressure as a prime risk factor for cardiovascular diseases. "High blood pressure" is exactly what it says—an increase in the pressure the heart has to exert to keep the blood pumping freely through our arteries. Naturally, nothing that puts a constant excessive work load on the heart could be good for us.

Although fewer women than men suffer from hypertension, the enormity of the problem dictates that we must all take it seriously, at any age. Thirty-two percent of American women between the ages of twenty-five and seventy-four have high blood pressure. It contributes to about one million deaths a year, affects 35 million people, and costs more than $15 billion in health expenditure annually.

If detected early, the condition is easily treated. Weight reduction and salt restriction alone are successful in reducing blood pressure to normal in about 25 percent of individuals with moderate hypertension. Exercise, stress reduction, and lifelong treatment with medications can greatly reduce the risk of diseases associated with hypertension, such as arteriosclerosis, heart attack, stroke, and kidney failure.

Recent statistics from the National Institutes of Health show that women between the ages of forty-five and seventy-four with elevated blood pressure have about twice the risk of developing clinical coronary heart disease. With that sobering thought, doesn't it make sense to keep your weight and blood pressure under control? Your physician should be monitoring your blood pressure on every visit you make to his office. If not, just ask him to check it; it takes only a few seconds and it could save your life.

## Reducing Your Risks

Nancy was forty-three when she felt what she thought were the first signs of impending cardiac doom. She had been on the train into New York City when she felt a dull but almost stabbing pain in her chest, just beneath her breastbone. As she walked from Grand Central Station to her midtown Manhattan office, she had to keep stopping to take a breather. The pain didn't last too long into the morning, but it was enough to send Nancy into a panic.

When Nancy called me from her office, she was almost in tears. "Dr. Shafto, this is going to sound weird, but I think I'm having a heart attack," she moaned.

I asked her to describe her symptoms in detail. Although it didn't sound like a full-blown heart attack, I was genuinely concerned because I knew from her family history that her father had suddenly dropped dead on the street from cardiac arrest at the age of fifty-two. I reassured my patient that what she had experienced was most probably not a heart attack but that she should be checked at the nearest hospital emergency room right away just to make certain.

Nancy's story is not unusual. Being an intelligent woman, she knew roughly what the symptoms of a heart attack were, but she still held fast to the old belief that women in their prime just don't die of heart attacks. That's why she sounded so confused and thought I would view her experience as "weird." Of course, the truth is that a heart attack can strike at any age, and, as we know, the risk for females greatly increases as they pass through their forties and fifties.

An electrocardiogram (EKG), which measures the electrical impulses of the heart, led the emergency-room doctors to believe that there was no imminent cause for concern. However, I had Nancy take the next day off from work to undergo a thorough workup in our hospital's cardiac unit. This included a stress test, exercising on a treadmill, which enables a physician to determine how efficiently the heart is functioning when it is under stress. In Nancy's case, her heart didn't do well when she was on the treadmill. The final diagnosis was not heart attack but angina pectoris. Although not deadly in itself, angina is a warning sign from the heart that it is not receiving enough oxygen to supply its needs under stress.

And Nancy was one of the typical working females who thought she thrived well under stress. Not content to work a ten- or eleven-hour day, she also took work home with her in the evenings. Combine that with her family history of heart disease, the fact that she'd been smoking a pack and a half of cigarettes for the past fourteen years (a habit I begged her to break when she came for her last major checkup five years ago), high blood pressure, and a high blood cholesterol level and you've got all the prime ingredients for one thing—a heart attack of major proportion.

191

The angina was indeed a blessing in disguise for Nancy, as it alerted her to the danger her heart was facing. The first step was to get her back on the road toward peak health—not an impossible task when prospective heart disease is caught in its earliest stages. This is where prevention, protection, and reducing the risk factors really count. We worked up a therapy regimen together, and Nancy really stuck to it. To lower her cholesterol, she followed a diet that was high in carbohydrates (don't anybody ever tell you they're fattening), slightly lower in protein, and greatly reduced in fats. She was prescribed medication—a simple fluid-retention-reducing diuretic—for her high blood pressure, and that was soon brought under control. In addition, she started on a regular exercise program that included both low-impact aerobics and a former love, tennis.

Within three months, Nancy had greatly lowered her risk from heart attack, felt fitter and more relaxed than she had in years, and, possibly because of a new sense of calm gained from a less stressful life-style, was able to quit smoking for good. She hasn't had any more angina, and, in fact, her latest exercise stress test showed her heart to have grown in its strength and ability to pump blood. If Nancy sticks to her healthier new life-style—and there's no reason to suspect that she won't—I think she can expect to stay at fairly low risk for angina and coronary artery disease, and be in good health for many years.

The secret with Nancy, as with many women our age, is that it's never too late to make a change for the better. It took a warning sign for Nancy, but for many of you a frank talk with your personal physician, a check over your family history, and a slight modification of your present life-style may be all that are needed to take out the most valuable insurance policy you can for the future well-being of your heart.

# Cholesterol

An increased level of cholesterol and other fats (lipids) in the blood is known to make coronary heart disease more likely. The atheromatous plaque I described on page 186 is partially composed of cholesterol. The tendency to have high cholesterol is sometimes inherited but increases with age and is mostly affected by diet. Many of us know this, but I will emphasize that a diet high in saturated fatty acids—found in red meat, animal fats, butter, whole milk and cream, cheese, and egg yolks—puts us at risk for heart attack. There has been a general tendency in recent years to follow a diet using more fruit and vegetables, whole grain cereals and breads, low-fat milk and cheese, fish and chicken and polyunsaturated vegetable oils, which is much more apt to keep the lipids at a normal level. Other lipids are important: women tend to have higher levels of HDL or high-density lipoproteins which protect against coronary artery disease by removing cholesterol from the circulation and assisting it to the liver which excretes it.[2] The liver does manufacture cholesterol even if we have none in our diet, as we do need some cholesterol (it is a building block in sex hormones and other hormones).

Obesity and smoking decrease the HDL (good-guy lipoprotein) and exercise increases it, so in order to decrease our risk for heart attack we should exercise regularly, never smoke, get down to our ideal weight, and follow a diet to keep our cholesterol level down and our HDL up. Normal levels of cholesterol are listed by laboratories in the following chart, but the American Heart Association recommends that the total cholesterol be kept below 200 mgm and the LDL (low-density lipoprotein, the bad-guy lipoprotein which carries cholesterol to the blood vessel walls to make the atheromatous plaque) below 125 mgm. The important number to know is your total cholesterol–HDL ratio, which is a good predictor for risk for heart attack. Total cholesterol measures the LDL cholesterol (usually two-thirds of total) plus HDL cholesterol plus VLDL (very low-density lipoproteins); the ratio is worked out from these numbers by dividing total cholesterol by the HDL. If you have ratios of 10 and 20 you are at double and triple the average risk, which is 5. If your ratio is 3 to 0 or less you are at an ideal level with low risk for atheromatous plaque formation. So at forty you should know your cholesterol level and your ratio and if you are at higher than normal risk you can do something about it. Triglycerides, other blood fats, are measured and should not run more than 60 mg/dl (range 40–180: ideal below 60). The triglyceride level is affected by food intake and is always measured fasting.

The Lipid Research Clinic Trials have shown that for every 1 percent reduction in cholesterol there was a 2 percent reduction in coronary heart disease.[3] So it really pays to keep your cholesterol low by reducing your dietary intake. The National Institutes of Health recommend all adults follow a diet which limits total fat to 30 percent of total calories and saturated fats to 10 percent of total calories and also reducing total calories to attain and maintain ideal body weight. If careful dieting and regular exercising do not result in acceptable cholesterol and ratio levels, there are drugs available but at our age we should be able to be in control without reverting to drugs which taste bad and have side effects. The role of fish oil in lowering triglycerides and VLDL is being researched and we will see the recommendations as they are made available in the press. Researchers have found that taking 4 to 6 grams of eicosapentenoic acid (EPA) daily lowers triglycerides 50 to 85 percent in normal people and in those with genetic problems of hypertriglyceridemia.[4]

Note that the "normal" levels that are printed out by laboratories for fatty acids, cholesterol, LDL, HDL, and triglycerides are average levels taken from people of varying ages in a population which is very prone in its older years to coronary heart disease. So plan on reaching and maintaining your levels in the low to normal range.

*Normal Cholesterol Levels in Women*

| | |
|---|---|
| Under age 20 | less than 180 mgm/dl |
| 20–40 | 140–240 |
| 41–50 | 150–280 |
| 50+ | 180–330 |

*HDL Levels and Risk Correlation*

| Serum HDL | Risk of Coronary Heart Disease (CHD) |
|---|---|
| 25 or less | very high risk |
| 26–35 | high risk |
| 36–44 | moderate risk |
| 45–59 | average risk |
| 60 or above | below average risk |

*Cholesterol–HDL Ratio Risk Prediction for CHD*

| | |
|---|---|
| 20 | very high risk |
| 10 | high risk |
| 5 | average risk |
| 3 | ideal: below average risk |

# CANCER

Cancer is second only to heart disease as the biggest killer among females. It is, however, the largest single cause of deaths among women aged thirty-five to fifty-four, according to the U.S. Department of Health and Human Services. You don't need to read between the lines to see that women our age are right in the middle of the cancer firing-line. Should this give us additional cause for alarm? Not if we use this information intelligently. To be forewarned is to be forearmed. I would like to be able to report a winning battle, but in general the mortality statistics remain about the same.

What is heartening, however, is that while the incidences of certain cancers remain the same or are growing, the survival rates are increasing every year, especially among victims of

195

breast cancer, the disease that strikes the most fear into the hearts of women at our time of life. One in eight women will develop cancer of the breast at some time during their life span and an estimated 40,000 American women eventually die of the dreaded disease each year. Yet, despite more cases of breast cancer being discovered, mostly due to widespread screening of asymptomatic women, increased female awareness, and superior techniques of detection, the mortality rate has dipped only very slightly. For example, the mortality rate from breast cancer in 1969 was 26.4 per 100,000 women; in 1980, 26 per 100,000. The good news is that the latest estimates for death rate from breast cancer hover around 18 percent. This downward trend is due mainly to the latest approaches to the treatment of breast cancer. Radiation therapy is most promising for women who have early-stage breast cancer. It is combined with surgery, but that surgery is far less radical than it was a decade ago. Only the lesion and a surrounding margin of breast tissue together with the underarm lymph nodes are removed before radiation treatment begins. At the National Cancer Institute (NCI), clinical trials are now comparing radiation's effectiveness with traditional surgical approaches, and the early findings look very encouraging. Already two projects are showing great promise for women with breast cancer. One indicates that there is a longer disease-free interval and improved survival rate for women receiving chemotherapy following mastectomy, and the second shows that monoclonal antibodies (genetically manipulated antibodies designed to hunt down specific cancers), when utilized as a detection tool to diagnose several forms of breast cancer, can provide the most sophisticated and sensitive early warning system yet devised for the detection of the disease.

Lung cancer is now perceived as the most devastating form of cancer we women face today. Although the incidence of this type of cancer is approximately a third that of breast cancer, the death rate has just recently surpassed breast cancer's by 2 percent and is currently estimated at 20 percent. It is presently the leading cause of cancer deaths among American women.

Colorectal cancer will strike 145,000 Americans this year, but it is one cancer that responds well to treatment if diagnosed early. Latest statistics indicate that it is the second leading incidence of cancer among women and the third highest in mortality rates. Most of the sixty thousand deaths could be avoided with the aid of simple tests that can detect the disease at a stage when it's 90 percent curable.

Cervical cancer also responds well to early treatment, with a 66 percent five-year survival rate for white females and 61 percent for black females. Research on cervical cancer and its causes is intense and several risk factors have been identified. The NCI is conducting an exhaustive study of two thousand women across the country in the hopes of arriving at a better understanding of this disease, its cause and epidemiology.

Fortunately early detection of cervical cancer is not only accurate but easily available with the sensitive Pap test and early therapy is often curative.

Cancer of the uterus, or endometrial cancer, is responsible for 9 percent of all female cancer deaths. Ovarian cancer claims more than eighteen thousand new victims each year, and eleven thousand lives. Studies at the NCI indicate that women who have been pregnant are half as likely to develop ovarian cancer as those who have not. There also appears to be a strong link between the development of breast and ovarian cancer. Those who have fallen prey to breast cancer are twice as likely to experience the growth of ovarian cancer, while victims of ovarian cancer are four times more likely to develop breast cancer.

# Cervical Cancer

I imagine there are very few of you who are not familiar with the Pap smear. It should be a regular part of your health checkup. Although many of you may be aware of the technique, you may not know how it actually works and its benefits.

197

The Pap test was developed in 1943 by Dr. George Papanicolau and became the most widespread early-detection system for cancer of the cervix. Considering its vital importance to us at our stage in life, it seems incredible that women over forty are three times less likely than women in their twenties and thirties to undergo regular Pap tests to detect cervical cancer. This neglect is all the more frightening because cancer of the cervix most often strikes older women. In fact, the number of cases begins to creep up alarmingly around the age of fifty and on into the sixties. The reason thousands of women either eliminate or reduce the frequency of their Pap smears as they approach middle age may be because of the conflicting recommendations coming from the American Cancer Society on one hand and the American College of Obstetricians and Gynecologists on the other. The Society recommends Pap smears every three years after two negative results, while the College calls for yearly examinations. There is no doubt in my mind that the benefits of the latter are obvious. Early detection most often means that cervical cancer can be successfully treated in a regular gynecological office visit, while delayed diagnosis can lead to costly hospital stays, expensive treatment, and surgery.

The Pap test, performed during an internal pelvic examination, is quite uncomplicated and painless and nothing to be apprehensive about. Using a small plastic or wooden spatula, your doctor scrapes some of the surface cells from the cervix and places them on a slide. This smear is then studied under the microscope to detect any early signs of abnormal cell growth.

## Interpreting Your Pap Score

So, you've just had your regular Pap test, the result is relayed from the lab to your doctor, and he gives you the news. The only problem is that it doesn't sound good. "The score wasn't normal. I think you'd better come back in and we'll have a second look," he says.

Don't panic. Such a finding does not mean you have cancer. What it does mean is that some abnormal cells were found on the cervical smear and, for safety's sake, it would be prudent to find out why these cells are there.

Remember that the Pap test is a screening tool and not a diagnostic test. It is there to sort the wheat from the chaff, to single out women who, for one reason or another, should have further testing. There are several ways of reporting a Pap-test result, based on counting the number and types of abnormal cells that show up when the test slide is examined under a microscope. The most common system divides the results into five different groups:

*Class I* indicates a negative or normal result. There is no suspicion or indication of cancer and nothing needs to be done except to repeat the test at the regular intervals you have already decided upon with your physician.

*Class II* indicates evidence of vaginal infection. This finding calls for the treatment of the infection and then a repeat Pap test to make sure the abnormal cells have disappeared and the Pap returns to Class I status.

*Class III* shows abnormal cellular changes that are most likely due to infection but that could also indicate the early stages of cancer.

*Class IV* reveals somewhat extensive abnormal cells and the likelihood that they are cancerous.

*Class V* indicates that cancer is present. Although the result is unquestionable for the presence of cancer cells, it gives no indication of how widespread the disease may be.

As a general rule, if I see a persistent Class II smear or a single incidence of Class III, IV, or V, I will immediately suggest further testing. This usually means a cervical biopsy, done under magnification under the colposcope, in the gynecologist's office. Colposcopy will permit the extent of the abnormal tissue to be identified: some lesions can be treated by removal with laser beam or cryotherapy in the office; others may need more extensive surgery, such as conization (a cone-sized piece of cervix is removed) or hysterectomy, in a hospital setting.

The greatest advantage of the Pap smear is that it can detect cervical cancer at its earliest stages, before it has time to spread and while it is still at its most vulnerable—and obviously its most curable. The test can also identify precancerous conditions that should also respond successfully to early treatment.

## BREAST CANCER

It's the one lump a woman dreads feeling—and with very good reason. At forty we should be more concerned than ever about breast cancer. The rate of cancer climbs during our thirties and goes on to hit its peak at menopause: about 20 percent of cases are diagnosed under the age of forty, and the average age of a woman when breast cancer is discovered is fifty-four. From then on, there is a little respite as the incidence levels out, but it is followed by a resurgence of increased cancer levels after the age of sixty-five.

So it is of paramount importance at our age that we take advantage of all the available screening devices for breast cancer, especially regular professional breast examinations, routine self-examinations, and the newly developed screening techniques for combating the disease.

But before we get deeply into breast cancer, remember one thing: not all lumps in the breast mean cancer. Go back to Chapter 6: there are significant other causes of lumps that are little cause for concern and certainly no indication for cancer worries; but a definitive diagnosis must be made.

The overall picture for breast cancer is not a pretty one. Breast cancer is the number-one cancer killer of women in the United States. A new case is diagnosed every thirteen minutes, and in 1985 the American Cancer Society predicted that the year would end with some 123,000 new cases of the disease: about 40,000 women die from breast cancer annually.

The biggest puzzle of breast cancer is that we have yet to positively identify its cause. Nobody knows for sure why there's a remarkably low incidence of breast cancer among Oriental women and a high incidence among women in Northern Europe. Genetic predisposition is the highest risk factor—increasing the chances of developing breast cancer sevenfold sometimes, especially if relatives develop the disease before menopause.

Risk factors for breast cancer:

- Age over forty (85 percent breast cancers forty+)
- Family history (mother or sister with breast cancer or other close relative)
- Early menarche (menses started before age twelve)
- First full-term pregnancy after thirty
- Never had children
- Previous surgery for benign breast disease
- Previous cancer of breast
- Previous cancer of uterus or ovary
- Obesity
- High-fat diet
- Caucasian (urban dweller)

Low risk for breast cancer:

- No family history
- Age under thirty
- Oriental
- First full-term pregnancy before age eighteen
- Surgical removal of ovaries before age thirty-seven

The mortality rate due to breast cancer has changed little since the 1950s; so, since we cannot prevent breast cancer as yet, the best method of attacking the problem is by early detection and treatment. If the cancer is limited to the breast, with treatment the survival rate over five years is better than 85 percent; but when the lymph nodes and peripheral areas are involved, that survival factor drops dramatically to 45 percent.

Clearly the greatest concern, once breast cancer has been diagnosed, is whether there is invasion of the lymph nodes. In practical terms, the more lymph nodes involved, the higher the chance of the condition becoming terminal.

Women who are in the very highest risk category are those who developed breast cancer during their twenties or thirties, as there is a 1 percent per year chance of developing cancer in the other breast.

## Self-Examination

As many as 80 percent of women discover their own breast tumors. And, thank goodness, the vast majority of these women don't wait around but report their findings to their physician or gynecologist immediately. It is this type of educated and intelligent response to the possibility of cancer that is saving the lives of female cancer victims today.

Examine your own breasts each month. The best time to do this is immediately after your period.

A lump in the armpit should never be ignored. It could be a swelling of the immune system's lymph nodes, indicating that your body is fighting something off, most probably an infection. But—and this is what makes reporting the condition to your physician crucial—a consistently swollen lymph node can often lead to the detection of cancer before a tumor can be felt in the breast.

Above all, remember that your first line of defense against breast cancer is as close as your own fingertips.

## Nipple Discharge

Most of my patients who are worried about cancer will see me after experiencing pain, discovering a mass, or noticing a discharge from a nipple. Nipple discharge, however, is not a common feature of breast cancer; only about 11 percent of women with discharge will have cancer. The phenomenon is

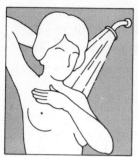

**1) IN THE SHOWER:**
Examine the entire area of each breast in the bath or shower, since fingers glide more easily over wet skin. Check for any lump or thickening.

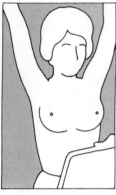

**2) BEFORE A MIRROR:**
Inspect your breasts first with arms overhead, and then by placing hands on hips and flexing your chest muscles. Look for any changes, i.e., dimpling or swelling.

**3) LYING DOWN:**
To examine your right breast, place a pillow or folded towel underneath your right shoulder and place your right hand behind your head. With left fingers flat, press each breast in small, circular motions around an imaginary clock face. Repeat for the left breast. Then, squeeze each nipple. Any discharge should be promptly reported to your physician. *American Cancer Society*®

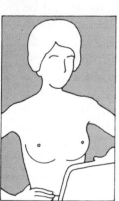

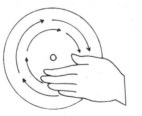

## SELF-TEST FOR BREAST CANCER DETECTION

203

quite common: the discharge can be milky, clear, or yellow in color and the causes of it are many. Usually it is stimulated by strenuous physical activity. Women who exercise heavily, especially on Nautilus equipment and other weight-training systems, often experience it. Birth-control pills and tranquilizers have also been linked with nipple discharge. A bloody discharge from the nipple should be investigated immediately, as should a discharge that forms a hard crusting, and possibly a secondary infection; the latter is often a sign of Paget's disease, which is a form of cancer. The general message with nipple discharge is: don't panic, but for your own self-assurance, always get it checked out by your physician or gynecologist.

## Latest Detection Techniques

Advances are being made every year in detecting breast cancer, greatly improving the chances of early detection for yourself. Mammography has been the workhorse of screening techniques for some years, and it's still considered by physicians to be the most reliable.

I'm often asked how often these diagnostic tests should be performed. For women up to the age of forty, I recommend an annual professional breast examination; for those over forty, examination twice a year. You may think my advice to be overly cautious, in light of the American Cancer Society's recommendation of an examination once every three years up to forty and once a year thereafter. I exercise caution because with today's superior detection techniques, there is little or no chance of any adverse side effects as a result of a thorough examinaton.

What follows is a review of mammography plus an update on the very latest techniques of detection.

***Mammography.*** Mammography uses low-level-dosage X rays to detect tissue changes that might not be apparent to the touch until one or two years down the road. The radiation controversy has made some women reluctant to undergo a mammogram, although the levels used today are less than a quarter of what was commonly used ten years ago, making the risk of hazards virtually nonexistent. If anything, the real risk lies in not having regular mammograms. A recent study from Sweden of more than 100,000 women indicated that mammography had resulted in a reduction of deaths due to breast cancer by 31 percent.

*Diaphanography.* In simple terms, this is a light scanning procedure in which white light is used to illuminate the breast tissue. Both malignant and benign tumors absorb light; a computer picks up the minute variations in light absorption and translates them into color images displayed on a monitor screen. Diaphanography is a safe, painless, and noninvasive (does not enter the body or put it at risk) technique that may have as high as a 90 percent accuracy rate, equal to that of mammography. In a 1983 study of 450 women, diaphanography detected fourteen malignant tumors, two of which were too small to be detected by hand and four that were missed by mammography. The technique may be particularly useful in screening pregnant women or women with particularly dense breast tissue, scar tissue, or silicone implants. This transillumination of the breast is currently used as an adjunct to physical examination and mammography.

*Thermography.* This technique has been used widely in Europe for the past twenty years, although feelings among health professionals in this country are mixed about its effectiveness. Because the temperature over a breast tumor is higher than that of surrounding healthy tissue, a "hot spot" may be detected at the surface of the skin. Thermography uses liquid crystals or a special film to detect hot spots, which can signify the need for further probing. The American College of Radiology has called the technique ineffective, but at least two large studies have shown the opposite to be true. When women without any discernible breast lumps who showed abnormalities on thermograms were given follow-up examinations, cancerous conditions *were* found. In one study, 33 percent of women who tested positive on thermograms did develop cancer within five years. The American Cancer Society and the National Cancer Institute decided after a trial of four years not to use thermography as a screening tool for breast cancer because of a lack of sensitivity and exactness in diagnosis.[5]

**Ultrasound.** This technique, also known as sonography, relies on sending pulsing, high-frequency sound waves into the breast. It is painless and noninvasive. The sound waves bounce back in an echo to a machine that interprets them in levels showing the density of tissues in the breast. The one drawback with ultrasound is that it has not been found to be particularly successful in detecting the smallest of lumps, which can obviously mean a crucial delay in early onset of treatment. It is, however, extremely useful in differentiating between benign and malignant growths—thus possibly eliminating the need for surgical biopsies. It is a very useful technique to differentiate between cystic and solid tumors and is used a lot in younger women as no radiation is involved.

**Nuclear magnetic resonance.** Also known as NMR, this diagnostic method uses a powerful magnet and radio waves to produce computer-enhanced cross sections of the breast. There are distinct advantages to this technique, which may make it the diagnostic test of choice among health professionals. It does not use potentially harmful forms of radiation, has no known side effects, and the cross-sectional representations of the breast are much easier to view than a whole picture. The technique has also been found to be highly successful in distinguishing between cancerous and noncancerous masses. Many proponents of NMR confidently predict that it will avert the need for an immediate surgical biopsy should a mammogram detect suspect tissue changes. One snag is that NMR does not pick up the microcalcifications which can be an early warning sign of cancer: it is very good for evaluation of lymph nodes.

# CT Scan

Computerized tomographic mammography, CTM, is a function of the CT (computerized axial tomography) scanner. Used to diagnose breast masses, it is of value when the mammogram is indeterminate; but it is costly and delivers a much larger dose of radiation to the entire chest. It is therefore not suitable for screening.

In conclusion, the best imaging for screening of breast cancer is generally agreed to be that of mammography, with ultrasound a useful adjunct to differentiate cystic from solid breast tumors. Other screening methods need further evaluation. Mammography requires 0.4 rad for xeromammography and 0.2 rad for screen-film mammography, compared with the slightly more than 1 rad required for CTM.

## Lowering the Risk Naturally

A recent study from Britain suggests that women who consume large amounts of Vitamin E might possibly have a lower risk of breast cancer. Researchers found significantly lower levels of the vitamin in the blood of a sample of thirty-nine women with known breast cancer than in that of seventy-eight women who were cancer-free. Women with the lowest levels of Vitamin E in their bloodstream had five times the risk of breast cancer than those with the highest levels of the vitamin. The researchers caution, however, that it is not known whether the deficiency of Vitamin E was a cause or an effect of the breast cancer. Another caveat: taking vitamin E may be associated with alterations in fatty acid or lipid metabolism. You should not take more than 400 IU daily.[6]

## Treatments

It used to be "Lose your breast or lose your life!" Not a very encouraging situation for any woman to face. Fortunately, there are alternatives to a radical mastectomy.

Today, mastectomy for breast cancer is thought to be both needlessly mutilating and actually insufficient by itself to be an effective form of totally eradicating cancer.

It is only in recent years that we have come to appreciate that breast cancer is not usually localized in the breast by the time it is diagnosed. Chances are the cancer has already migrated to distant organs or bones, even when it cannot be detected in the lymph glands closest to the affected breast. We also know that it can take some eight to ten years for a single tumor to grow large enough to be detected, and even the most aggressive cancer takes at least three years to grow from a single cell to the size of a small grape, when it might first become detectable as a lump.

The growing trend in the United States is toward a less radical approach to combating breast cancer. There are a number of treatments to choose from. Today, the most common is a lumpectomy, which requires the removal of the tumor mass and surrounding tissue but essentially leaves the breast cosmetically intact. The next step is to hit any remaining cancer cells (including those that have wandered to other parts of the body) with radiation therapy.

A recent study from Italy tends to support the move away from radical surgery. Out of 701 breast-cancer patients studied, long-term survival rates among women who had a traditional radical mastectomy and those who had a quadrantectomy (an operation that removes only the tumor and a quarter of the breast) followed with radiation therapy were almost identical. The Harvard Joint Center for Radiation Therapy recommends that, ideally, lumpectomy plus radiotherapy could be appropriate treatment for up to 85 percent of all breast-cancer victims.

Unfortunately, in almost half of all breast cancers diagnosed in this country each year, cancer cells will have already migrated to other parts of the body. There's good news, though, in the form of the new anticancer drugs. In one recent study, the use of a combination of drugs in chemotherapy has meant better than a five-year survival rate for nearly 80 percent of younger women and 75 percent of postmenopausal women who developed breast cancer.

Another large-scale study offers new hope for older women who have a type of breast cancer that is particularly sensitive to estrogen. Following surgery, doctors gave half the women anticancer drugs along with a drug called tamoxifen, which blocks the action of estrogen; the control group received the chemotherapy without the estrogen-blocking drug. The women who received tamoxifen had up to 64 percent fewer cancer recurrences in the first two years following detection than did those in the control group.

# LUNG CANCER

The most serious news in the cancer field is that lung cancer has now overtaken breast cancer as the number-one cancer killer among American women. The death rate for women who develop lung cancer is 20 percent for those diagnosed in recent years, compared with about 18 percent for those diagnosed with breast cancer. Breast cancer still has a higher incidence than lung cancer among women; it will affect 27 percent of the female population, whereas lung cancer will affect 11 percent.

While early diagnosis and more aggressive treatments for breast cancer have stemmed fatalities, that has not been the case with lung cancer. The rising lung-cancer death rate is due to increased incidence and lack of effective therapy. Smoking has been determined to be the overwhelming factor affecting the incidence rate.

The lungs, however, do have an amazing ability to repair injury. If you stop smoking when you are forty, much of the accumulated tar can be removed by your lungs' natural cleansing system. Rupture of the dividing walls, or septa, of the alveoli—the air sacs in the lungs—is related to age and happens gradually to us all. But people who have never smoked have emphysema to a much lesser degree than do smokers. In smokers, emphysema is always present after a time and increases with age and the degree of exposure to tobacco smoke. Emphysema, the rupture of tiny alveolar walls that causes the lungs to have fewer larger air sacs instead of many tiny ones, interferes with breathing and the amount of oxygen available to the lungs as the surface area of the lung decreases in this way. The symptoms are shortness of breath, cough, reduced tolerance for exercise, and heavy breathing. Emphysema is a major cause of chronic pulmonary disease and may lead to heart failure.

Rare before the age of thirty, lung cancer is most common in the fifties and sixties—and is ten to thirty times more common in smokers. Of those who smoke for forty years, 4 percent will develop lung cancer. The death rate from this disease increases fourfold with advancing years in the nonsmoker, but the risk of developing the disease is ten times greater in the smoker.

Not all lung tumors are malignant: if a chest X ray indicates that you have a tumor you have a 5 percent chance that it will be benign.

Exposure to industrial chemicals affects men more than it does women: chronic obstructive diseases of the lungs are common, but, again for example, 14 percent of asbestos workers who smoke will develop lung cancer—obviously a higher rate than the cancer risk among smokers not exposed to asbestos.

The picture is clear. More young women are smoking than ever before, and the projected rates of emphysema and lung-cancer development are frighteningly high. The longer you smoke, the worse the *final* picture will be. If you stop smoking now that you are forty you have an excellent chance that your risk for developing and dying from cancer, coronary artery disease, and chronic lung disease will be enormously reduced. Consider those facts when you go to buy your next pack of cigarettes.

# COLON CANCER

It's the cancer women don't talk about; yet women over forty are at highest risk for this disease. Surveys show that most of us are reluctant to talk about it even with our doctors. Believe it or not, only one in four women ever asks her physician to examine their colon or rectum.

Yet colon and rectal cancer are 90 percent curable if detected early, and the five-year survival rate for these cancers has improved over the past few decades to slightly more than 50 percent for all cases of colon cancer whether detected early or late.

Three tests are recommended by the American Cancer Society (ACS) for the early detection of colon and rectal cancer before obvious symptoms become apparent: after forty, have an annual digital rectal exam in which the physician feels inside the rectum with a gloved finger; every year after age fifty, a stool-blood-slide test, which identifies any hidden blood, and at intervals a proctosigmoidoscopy, which allows the physician to inspect the rectum and lower colon with a rigid lighted tube.

Recent medical findings indicate that the site of most colorectal cancers is shifting higher in the colon, so longer, flexible lighted instruments have been developed which allow the physician to view the entire rectum and colon and remove any polyps at the same time. The flexible colonoscope is much better tolerated than the proctosigmoidoscope. The ACS recommends a colonoscopy every three to five years after age fifty, following two annual normal exams. If any of these tests reveals possible problems, a barium enema X ray with air contrast to examine in detail the gastrointestinal tract will probably be performed.

Mistaken notions about the tests and the disease abound:

- It is commonly thought that a negative stool test in a woman approaching fifty eliminates the need for a rectal or sigmoidoscopy or colonoscopy exam. Wrong. All

211

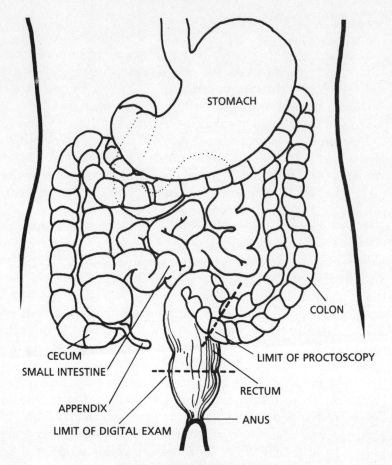

STOMACH

COLON

CECUM
SMALL INTESTINE

LIMIT OF PROCTOSCOPY

APPENDIX

RECTUM

LIMIT OF DIGITAL EXAM

ANUS

## THE DIGESTIVE TRACT

This illustration shows the limits to which a physician's digital and proctoscope examinations can detect cancer. *National Cancer Institute* three tests may be necessary for a thorough, conclusive evaluation.

- The disease does not strike more men than women; the reverse is true.
- A popular misconception is that surgical treatment will result in a permanent colostomy, an artificial opening in the abdominal wall to permit elimination of waste. In fact, a permanent colostomy is seldom needed, owing to advances in surgical techniques. Chemotherapy is now being studied as a viable alternative to a colostomy in advanced cases.

Women in our age range should take special care to watch for a number of warning signs. These include rectal bleeding, blood in the stool, and any marked change in bowel habits. There are risk factors, too, that we should all be aware of:

- Family history of colorectal cancer
- Family history of familial polyposis or presence of polyps in the colon
- Previous inflammatory bowel disease or ulcerative colitis
- Presence of polyps in the colon (benign adenomas may contain malignant tissue)
- High-fat and low-fiber diet
- Advancing age

We have become a nation of high-fat, low-fiber eaters, which significantly increases our risk of colon cancer. It is wise to reduce the amount of fat in our diet and increase consumption of cereals, fresh fruits, and vegetables.

# CANCER OF THE CERVIX

Cancer of the cervix is one cancer that has actually declined markedly over the past decade. The disease presently affects

8.8 cases per 100,000 among white females, but in comparison a much higher 20.2 cases among black females. The five-year survival rate for cervical cancer stands at 66 percent for whites and 61 percent for blacks.

No primary cause has yet been positively identified for cervical cancer. However, the highest incidence of the disease occurs among women who first started having intercourse early in their teens and who have continued to be sexually active over the years with multiple partners. (Frequency of intercourse is not suspected, as the same high risk is not apparent among women who have very frequent intercourse with one long-term partner.) All signs indicate that cervical cancer may have a strong link to the incidence of venereal disease, especially herpes virus and papilloma virus infections.

Gynecologists are now able to spot the earliest stages of cervical cancer—often years before a Pap smear can detect it. The secret is a simple, relatively inexpensive ($2,500) camera called a cerviscope. If researchers working with the new technique are correct, it could give us the best-ever chance of beating the cancer that strikes fourteen thousand American women a year.

In one major study reported at this year's annual meeting of the American College of Obstetricians and Gynecologists, the cerviscope was found to be far more accurate than the Pap smear. More than 3,200 women were tested with both Pap smears and the cerviscope. The cerviscope was over four times more sensitive in the detection of precancerous changes, finding fifty-four suspect lesions while the Pap smear could find only twelve. The results were later confirmed by colposcopy—a highly accurate diagnostic procedure that is impractical for mass screening because of its cost. In a study at Detroit's Sinai Hospital, 1,400 women were screened, with the Pap smear displaying a false negative rate of 64 percent compared with just 20 percent for the cerviscope.

Developed at the Medical College of Wisconsin, the camera is able to detect microscopic changes in the tissue and blood vessels of the cervix, where telltale signs indicate that cancer is developing. By diagnosing the cancer at such an early stage, the cerviscope offers the patient a far greater chance of beating the disease with immediate treatment. The Wisconsin physicians estimate that the cost of a cerviscope reading will be as little as $15 to $25, about as much as the present Pap test. Because of its greater accuracy and reliability, it could mean a test for most women only once every five years.

The cerviscope works by using a bright light to photograph the cervix through the vagina. Film is then sent to a laboratory, where the slide, or cervigram, is developed and magnified sixteen to twenty-five times on a screen. It is then carefully evaluated by specially trained physicians, and the results are sent to the patient's gynecologist. It takes approximately two weeks for the patients to get the results, whereas the Pap-smear results take about one week. So far, around 25,000 American women have been tested with the cerviscope, and it is being used in over 200 institutions and doctors' offices. Recommendations for a cerviscopic examination are every five years up to the age of forty-five. At that age the pertinent tissues and blood vessels move slightly, so they cannot be viewed by the camera lens: interval Pap smears are advised after that. The Wisconsin researchers say that having a cerviscopic exam in addition to a routine Pap smear will reduce the chances of a woman developing an undetected cancer to extremely remote levels. Eventually, after the cerviscope has been more widely tested, it is likely to become the routine diagnostic test for cervical cancer. The American Cancer Society advises that while the cerviscope may be a very important advance in the early detection of cervical cancer, women should not abandon the Pap test altogether.

Precancerous changes can occur in the tissue and blood vessels of the cervix up to ten years before the cancer starts to become life-threatening. Once they're detected, the cervix is usually treated by destroying the affected cells with cauterization or freezing.

# UTERINE AND OVARIAN CANCER

Fortunately uterine, or endometrial, cancer is relatively easy to detect and consequently shows a very high survival rate: 87 percent of white women and 54 percent of black women will live five years or more after detection. Why the disparity? According to the U.S. Department of Health and Human Services, this may be because of later detection among black women. You know by now what to ask me: what are the risk factors? What are the warning signs?

Risk factors for endometrial cancer are:

- Advancing age
- Family history of uterine cancer
- History of breast or colon cancer
- Obesity
- Polycystic ovary disease
- Nulliparity (never having had children)
- Menopausal women treated with estrogen without concomitant progesterone

The warning symptoms are irregular bleeding between periods at any age (only 5 percent of cases of uterine cancer occur before age forty) and any bleeding at all in postmenopausal women. There are benign causes of postmenopausal bleeding but it is crucial to assume it may be caused by cancer and to have testing done. The Pap test may occasionally show up some abnormal cells from the uterus but is basically not a screening test for endometrial cancer. The standard test is either a dilatation and curettage or an endometrial biopsy to obtain tissue for examination (see page 98) and sometimes a hysterosalpingogram (see page 97) or hysteroscopy (direct vision of the endometrium through an instrument passed through the cervix). The most heartening news about uterine cancer is a recent report from the National Center for Disease Control, which states that long-term use of the Pill may reduce the risk of endometrial cancer.

Ovarian cancer, which claims nearly twenty thousand new victims a year, has a five-year survival rate of 34 percent for white women and 35 percent for black women. Recent studies at the National Cancer Institute are offering some interesting new clues as to the prevention of ovarian cancer. Researchers have discovered that women who have been pregnant at least once are half as likely to develop the disease as women who have never been pregnant. And the greater the number of pregnancies attained, the lower the chances of contracting ovarian cancer. Even more interesting: women who have taken the Pill have been found to have a 10 to 50 percent reduced risk of ovarian cancer. Why? The Pill creates a hormonal balance similar to that found in pregnancy!

One of the most interesting recent developments in the early detection of ovarian cancer is not a new-fangled gadget or machine but some very ordinary, easily recognizable warning signals that every woman of our age should note. Until now, the lethal tumors were thought to produce no symptoms until well advanced. However, researchers at the University of Iowa recently identified telltale early signs that are experienced by almost 80 percent of women with cancer of the ovaries. Yet these signs have hitherto been largely ignored by women as inconsequential.

Doctors now believe that by making all of us aware of the subtle changes linked to the disease, more will seek early treatment and the eleven thousand deaths a year will be cut dramatically. I consider it an extremely important discovery, as statistics on survival rate for this disease are quite dismal—37 percent. This terrible picture occurs because ovarian cancer is usually not discovered until it has spread to other parts of the body. With early detection, however, the cure rate leaps to over 85 percent, meaning a far greater potential for saving more lives now that early-warning symptoms have been identified.

Nearly one hundred women—all newly diagnosed—took part in the unique Iowa study. In one-third, the cancer was confined to the ovaries; in the rest, it had spread. They were questioned extensively about their medical history and any physical changes that may have occurred in the months prior to diagnosis. The researchers found that certain conditions were reported time and again and they were able to establish these as definite symptoms of the cancer:

- Abdominal swelling
- Fatigue
- Abdominal pain
- Urination problems (frequency, difficulty, or discomfort)
- Irregular vaginal bleeding
- Uterine bleeding in postmenopausal women

Almost 80 percent of those with early disease experienced one or more of these symptoms, but the majority of the women who took part in the study had delayed seeking medical attention because they were unaware the changes could mean cancer. In fact, fewer than one-fifth said they'd felt concerned, and then not enough to see a doctor.

Ovarian cancer grows rapidly, so any delay in seeking treatment can prove costly in terms of survival. Tumors develop rapidly, quickly invading both ovaries. Malignant cells are also released from tumors earlier than with other cancers, mostly deposited on nearby organs like the bowel, bladder, and uterus—so within a few months the cancer is spreading around the body. Equally important, there are no screening tests for ovarian cancer; thus the discovery of early warning signals is a major advance.

It should be noted that many of the symptoms also occur with other, far less serious conditions. Painful urination, for example, can mean an infection in the bladder or the urethra, which carries urine from the bladder; irregular vaginal bleeding may simply be caused by changing birth-control pills; and fatigue may be the result of stress. But if any of these symptoms persist for a week—especially if you're suffering more than one symptom—and you have no plausible explanation, I advise you to see your physician and insist on a pelvic examination as part of the evaluation. Don't let it go longer than a week. If it does turn out to be cancer, there's a good chance your persistence and awareness of the warning symptoms will significantly improve the likelihood of a cure.

# AIDS

Acquired Immunodeficiency Disease, or AIDS, is an illness which was first described in the early 1980s and is now spreading throughout the world. AIDS is characterized by loss of the human body's normal fighting-off capacity or immunity to infections and unusual types of cancers which can then prove to be lethal.

- Acquired: this condition is not carried by genes and is therefore not inherited. It is not caused by either legal or illegal drugs.
- Immuno: the body has a built-in system to protect itself from infection and disease—the immune system: AIDS destroys this system.
- Deficiency: a lack of immunity which is a fatal problem.
- Syndrome: a group of signs and symptoms which collectively indicate a disease or abnormal condition.

While AIDS is found among all the following high-risk groups, it is spreading to the sexual partners of the first four groups:

- Gay or bisexual men (64 percent)
- Gay or bisexual IV drug users (8 percent)

219

- Heterosexual male and female IV drug users (17 percent)
- Recipients of blood or blood products (especially hemophiliacs who need multiple blood product infusions—3 percent)
- Heterosexual transmission (4 percent)
- Children under thirteen (usually infected by the mother during pregnancy or before and after birth—1 percent)

These statistics apply to 97 percent of AIDS cases in the United States. In other parts of the world men and women are equally affected and transmission may be mostly through heterosexual contact with body fluids.

In the United States the incidence in females is increasing, although mostly in women in contact with the abovementioned high-risk groups.

AIDS is caused by a virus which has several names; the most commonly used is HIV, Human Immunodeficiency Virus. Other names are HTLV-III, Human T cell Lymphotrophic Virus Type III; ARV, AIDS-Related Virus; and LAV, Lymphadenopathy-Associated Virus.

HIV virus has been proven to be transmitted by sexual contact which permits the exchange of semen or blood: injection of legal blood products or illegal virus-containing blood in IV drug users who share needles, and by passage of the virus to fetus or newborn by the infected mother. While HIV has also been found in saliva, tears, breast milk, urine, and vaginal secretions, transmission is very uncommon through these body fluids. Saliva sprayed in a cough or sneeze or left on a drinking glass has not been implicated in a case of AIDS. As blood for blood transfusion is now screened for the virus, this will no longer be a route of transmission but people who received blood before screening was widespread (between 1979 and 1985) may be at risk. Blood donation is, and always has been, absolutely safe for the donor.

Cases among women are increasing: women who have had sexual relationships with bisexual men or intravenous drug users may be at risk for AIDS. The statistics as of 1986 reveal that 7 percent of all cases of AIDS are in women. Of those, 50 percent were IV drug users, 27 percent contracted the disease by sexual contact with HIV-infected men, 10 percent had received contaminated blood or blood products, and 11 percent were of undetermined cause.

The most common warning signs of AIDS are:

- Fever for more than ten days, unexplained
- Swollen lymph nodes (glands) for more than three months, unexplained
- Prolonged fatigue, not caused by other medical or emotional conditions
- Diarrhea, persistent and severe
- Coughs, colds, and sore throats lasting for several weeks in nonsmokers
- Night sweats, drenching
- Thrush of the mouth (thick white dry coating)
- Recent appearance of purple lesions of the skin which increase in size
- Bruising easily or bleeding for inadequate reasons
- Weight loss (more than 10 percent of body weight, unexplained)

Many of these symptoms may be caused by other minor ailments or, for example, infectious mononucleosis, but if you are concerned and these problems are lasting and unexplained, see your doctor.

The infections and cancers which cause death in people whose immunity is suppressed are numerous and characteristic: the most common are pneumocystis carinii pneumonia, Kaposi's sarcoma (cancer), and various kinds of meningitis.

There is no treatment for AIDS: the various opportunistic infections and malignancies are treated as they arise. Research

221

is aimed at finding drugs to control HIV and to prevent infection by developing a vaccine. This will take a long time and will be announced in the press when available, so our best bet is to educate the general population, including adolescents, in methods of prevention by reducing exposure to the virus. This means changing behavior—in particular, sexual behavior. Clearly, abstinence is the safest sexual behavior, or a committed monogamous relationship with a faithful partner, but if these are not followed then careful use of a condom reduces the chance of passage of the virus from semen to the blood stream in vaginal or anal intercourse when often small abrasions occur. Just as the condom is not 100 percent effective in preventing pregnancy, it is not infallible in preventing AIDS and must be used with extreme care. Completely safe sex includes any activity where body fluids are not exchanged. High-risk sexual behavior includes vaginal intercourse with ejaculation in the presence of small abrasions; anal intercourse similarly, when the rectal mucosa is often torn; and oral sex. (Small lacerations of the mouth can be caused by toothbrushing.)

Avoiding blood-to-blood transmission means not doing intravenous drugs, especially with shared needles and other equipment.

This is all very frightening, isn't it? But remember: if you have no contact with high-risk groups you are not likely to be exposed. What is difficult is that people may not be truthful about, for instance, being bisexual. Know your partner well and talk about these concerns. It is clear that casual sex is now extremely dangerous—practice safe sex and protect yourself. With the high divorce rate in the United States and in other countries, women certainly have to be concerned as they seek another partner. But don't become panic-stricken about AIDS. Remember that men of your generation are also concerned and should be willing to exercise extreme caution in a relationship. I have heard younger people in their twenties say that they are not going to worry and will just "wing it," but you are not twenty-five and you understand the value of life and that this is a disease that kills. So you will be careful.

About testing for AIDS: testing is available at many hospitals and public health departments. It is often anonymous, with only a number used for identification. A positive test means only that you have been exposed to the virus and have made antibodies against it. You may be infected with the virus and may be contagious. You do not know from a positive test that you have AIDS or ARC (AIDS-Related Complex, a milder illness which may or may not go on to AIDS) or whether you will develop either condition later. Also, a negative test means only that your body has not made antibodies against HIV at the time of the testing: there is a "window" between being infected with the virus and the presence of detectable antibodies in the bloodstream; this means that the test turns positive after an interval. For these reasons it is usual for counseling to be offered before and after testing to evaluate risk factors and advise on your behavior in the future. As you know, there are major problems with confidentiality and discrimination issues related to HIV testing.

Hotlines are readily available in most large cities and information is available at public health agencies.[7]

Scientists spearheading AIDS research are constantly producing new and updated facts on this serious disease, setting out the latest guidelines for prevention and protection while they work to develop a vaccine against AIDS. My best advice to you is to be very careful in your sexual behavior and keep abreast of the ever-changing picture through your local press, TV newscasts, or medical and health magazines. Be knowledgeable about AIDS and its means of transmission and prevention: AIDS is not someone else's problem anymore.

# 8

# Food for Thought

The first time I heard "You are what you eat," I couldn't help but chuckle. But the more I thought about it, the more I realized just how true it is. After all, our entire bodies are made up of chemicals, and they don't just appear out of thin air. There's no magic compound that we draw from to supply the cells of our body with the energy they constantly need. And we don't have the ability to manufacture the majority of chemical elements we need. So, where do we get them?

Our foods supply all the chemicals we need. Like tinkertoys, our bodies break down the individual chemicals and rebuild them into the building blocks of life. When constructing a building, if you are not getting the right sand for the mortar or the correct clay for the bricks, the entire structure can fall apart. That's exactly what happens when we fail to supply our bodies with the nutrients they need.

# BALANCED DIET

I cannot stress enough the importance of a balanced diet for women at our age. All a balanced diet means is getting the intake of protein, carbohydrate, and fat into good equilibrium, so there's no reason why you can't benefit from the knowledge of what this proper equilibrium is.

For years we were told that we should all be eating mountains of protein and steering clear of fats and carbohydrates. If only we'd known then what we know now! According to the latest findings in nutritional science, we couldn't have been more wrong. While we've been consuming massive amounts of meat, we've been increasing our risk of heart and blood-vessel disease and colon cancer—to name a few problems associated with high intake of saturated fats and cholesterol. Meanwhile we've been ignoring the carbohydrates that contain the energy we need to fight back against ill health and disease, and avoiding the roughage and fiber necessary to keep the bowels regular and sidestep problems like colon cancer. To be honest, over the past four decades, we've been doing just about everything possible to abuse our bodies nutritionally!

Many of us used to get much of our protein from meat sources, with red meats being the most popular. There are two major problems here: first, red meats, no matter how lean they look, can have a fat content as high as 60 percent; and second, we eat about three times as much meat protein as our bodies really need. The result of years on this type of diet: high cholesterol and obesity. The recommended protein intake for a mature female is forty-two grams per day—or approximately the same amount of protein that would be supplied in six ounces of meat. You'd get almost all the protein you need in one quarter-pound burger. Anything more than that and you are putting an unnecessary strain on your digestive system. If the body has no use for the excess protein, it has to go somewhere—either stored away as reserve energy in fat

cells or excreted through the digestive tract. Additional unnecessary protein also puts a greater strain on the liver, whose
job, in simple terms, is to break down the chemical constituents
of all foods, sort what is needed and what isn't, and detoxify
any compounds that the body may find toxic.

Remember you were always told that carbohydrate foods—
pastries, pastas, potatoes, breads—would make you fat? Well,
it's just not so. Carbohydrates, more than any other food source,
supply the body with readily available energy. Which do you
think contains more calories, a lean three-ounce steak or three
ounces of spaghetti? Surprise, surprise! The steak contains
five hundred calories, the spaghetti three hundred. Only the
fat content in pastries and breads is going to add on the pounds,
certainly *not* the carbohydrates contained in them. Low-calorie
(or fat-reduced) breads and sweets are now widely available,
so why not take advantage of them and give your body an
energy boost.

We need very little fat in our daily diets, but that small
amount is essential to aiding the body's chemical conversions.
Latest nutritional findings indicate that no more than 30 percent of our total caloric intake should be fat. At the moment,
the average American daily consumption of fat is closer to 45
percent or more. The only fats we need are polyunsaturated
fats, since we can create saturated fats in our own bodies. That
is what body fat is: polyunsaturated fat that has been stored
as saturated fat in the body! We can obtain polyunsaturated
fats from oils in such plants as corn, peanut, safflower, and
soya. They are also found in cold-water fish. We can get
these fats directly from the source; we can also receive them
"second hand" in meats. The animal has already converted the
polyunsaturated fats (from the plant produce it ate) into saturated fat, which it stores in its tissues. Unfortunately, when
we eat meat, we also receive the animal's own saturated fats,
which we *don't* need. It's interesting to note that all our daily
fat needs could be supplied by one tablespoon of safflower
oil.

# The Ideal Balance

The ideal balanced diet recommended by leading nutritionists today is far removed from that of two or three decades ago. It's as simple as this: of your daily food intake, 12 percent should be protein, 58 percent carbohydrates, and 30 percent fats. This balance is now highly lauded by the American Heart Association, the American Cancer Society, and the National Institutes of Health.

Here, courtesy of Dr. Robert L. Pollack, professor of nutrition and biochemistry at Temple University, Philadelphia, and author of *The Pain-Free Diet,* are three days' worth of sample menus that correspond to this ideal protein-carbohydrate-fat balance. Each day provides 1,500 calories:

**Day 1:** *Breakfast:* 1 cup pineapple or orange juice, 1 egg (poached or boiled), 1 slice whole-grain toast, 1 teaspoon margarine, 1 cup skim milk. *Lunch:* ½ cup tuna (packed in water), 2 slices bread, 4 teaspoons mayonnaise, ½ cup tomato juice, 1 medium apple. *Dinner:* lettuce (as much as wanted), 2 teaspoons Roquefort dressing, 3 oz. baked chicken (without skin), ½ cup peas, ½ cup mashed potatoes, 2 plums, ½ cup skim milk. *Bedtime snack:* 4 graham crackers, ½ cup skim milk.

**Day 2:** *Breakfast:* 1 cup grapefruit juice, 1 bagel, ¼ cup cottage or cream cheese, 1 cup skim milk. *Lunch:* 1½ oz. cold cuts, 1 teaspoon mayonnaise, 2 slices bread, 2 teaspoons margarine, lettuce to garnish. *Dinner:* lettuce, 1 tablespoon dressing, 3 oz. lean hamburger, 1 roll, ½ cup spaghetti, ½ cup carrots, ½ cup bean sprouts, 1 peach, ½ cup skim milk. *Bedtime snack:* 1 piece angel or sponge cake, ½ cup skim milk.

**Day 3:** *Breakfast:* 1½ cups cereal, 4 teaspoons raisins, 6 small nuts, 1 cup skim milk. *Lunch:* Turkey sandwich, 2 slices whole wheat bread, lettuce, ½ cup tomatoes, 1 tea-

spoon mayonnaise, 1 medium orange. *Dinner:* ½ cup mashed
potatoes or yams, ½ cup cabbage, ½ cup green beans, 3
oz. baked sole, ½ cup peas, 1 large tangerine, ½ cup skim
milk. *Bedtime snack:* 1½ cups popcorn (no-salt, no-fat), ½
cup skim milk.

## SPECIAL VITAMIN AND MINERAL NEEDS

As women we do have to take into account additional nutritional needs, not necessarily because we are in our forties,
but for sound all-round health reasons.

*Anemia.* A good, varied diet should provide twelve milligrams of iron per two thousand calories, which is enough for
males and postmenopausal women. Between 5 and 10 percent
of iron is actually absorbed (about 0.6 to 1.2 milligrams), and
the minimum daily requirements are between 0.5 and 1 mil-
ligram per day. For those of us who are eating less than two
thousand calories a day and who are still menstruating, this
intake of iron is barely adequate. I suggest you supplement
your diet with iron-rich foods, such as red meat, liver, eggs,
whole-grain breads, cereals, and green vegetables. If this does
not bring the level of iron in the blood to normal (40 percent
of women between thirty and fifty display some degree of
anemia), I recommend supplemental iron: five to ten milligrams in capsule or tablet form.

An interesting little-known side benefit of oral contraception is that, as menstruation is usually much lighter for women
on the Pill, there's less iron-deficiency anemia.

*Urinary tract infections (UTIs).* If you are susceptible to
urinary infections, you can lower the risk by drinking a glass
or two of cranberry juice a day, which aids in making urine
more acidic. Urinary tract bacteria thrive more in an alkaline
environment.

*Premenstrual depression.* Increased estrogen levels immediately before your period can suppress the activity of vitamin $B_6$, which in turn compromises the ability of the amino acid tryptophan to build the all-important brain chemical serotonin. Latest research indicates that serotonin plays a key role in regulating sleep, pain, appetite, and, yes, depression! A daily supplement of fifteen to twenty milligrams of $B_6$ and ten milligrams of niacin should help. A daily booster dose of five hundred milligrams of tryptophan can also be added. All these nutritional supplements are readily available over the counter in pharmacies, supermarkets, and health-food stores. (See Premenstrual Syndrome, page 139.)

*Premenstrual bloating.* As estrogen and progesterone levels rise, we tend to retain salt and water. A week before menstruation, try to cut back on your regular salt and caffeine intake.

*Contraceptive pill.* Because we already know that higher levels of estrogen affect $B_6$ metabolism, I suggest to my patients on the Pill that they might want to consider taking $B_6$ supplements if they notice any abnormal fatigue or depression.

*Pregnancy.* I recommend that my patients increase their protein intake by about one ounce per day and make sure they drink between four and five glasses of skim milk to supply additional calcium. It's also a good idea to take a multivitamin supplement that contains all the necessary RDAs to ensure that you don't sustain any dietary deficiencies. Iron supplements may also be taken, but not more than twenty milligrams a day.

*Breast-feeding.* We need more calories, as much as one thousand a day, than when not breast-feeding. I also suggest increasing those four or five glasses of milk you were taking during pregnancy to about six or seven glasses. You will need to drink extraordinary amounts of fluid to keep up your milk production. Most women lose weight easily when nursing a baby!

*Sleep problems.* The old standby has always been milk. Here's something else to try. Tryptophan, the important natural amino acid we talked about earlier, helps control sleep. About forty-five minutes before retiring, take a five hundred-milligram tablet or capsule of tryptophan with a glass of orange juice or a high-carbohydrate snack.

# FOODS AND DRUGS THAT DON'T MIX

We all know that a variety of foods are essential to our good health. And drugs, too, are necessary at times to prevent and treat illness. However, some food and drug combinations can spell trouble. It's as well to be aware that certain foods can lower the effectiveness of some medications, and in a smaller number of cases actually result in adverse effects that can be dangerous and even fatal.

Unwanted and unexpected food and drug interactions can occur at any time of life, and as our bodies become older, we may become more susceptible to these chemical reactions. By knowing which food-drug combinations to avoid, you can protect your own good health and that of your family as well.

Tetracycline is a commonly prescribed antibiotic used to treat bacterial infections. Its effectiveness can be greatly reduced when it is taken with dairy products. Certain nutrients—for example, calcium, magnesium, aluminum, and iron—bind to the tetracycline, thus interfering with its absorption and preventing its medicinal action. Calcium is found in milk, cheese, yogurt, and other dairy products; iron-rich foods include red meat and dark-green vegetables; and magnesium and aluminum are found in commonly taken antacids. If your physician prescribes tetracycline, take it on an empty stomach, one hour before or two hours after a meal. If stomach upsets require you to take it with foods, make sure they do not contain dairy products.

A prime example of a beverage that can exaggerate a drug's desired effect is alcohol, which interacts with certain drugs and can pose a lethal threat to health. The effects of tranquilizers, barbiturates, painkillers, and antihistamines are all intensified when taken with alcohol, or if alcohol is consumed during their peak absorption periods. The combination can slow down mental and physical performance skills and judgment. Some drugs, especially anticonvulsants, work in reverse: the effect of both the alcohol and the drug is heightened. As a rule of thumb, just to be on the safe side, never take alcohol when you are on any prescription medication.

Another drug interaction occurs between a class of drugs known as monoamine oxidase inhibitors (MAO)—most often prescribed for depression—and foods that contain tyramine, a chemical found mainly in wine, beer, yogurt, chocolate, and cheeses. The body normally converts tyramine into a harmless, inactive compound, but in the presence of MAO inhibitors it converts to norepinephrine, a powerful brain chemical that can constrict blood vessels. As a result, blood pressure can suddenly skyrocket, and an unsuspecting victim can quickly become light-headed, dizzy, and even develop excruciating headache and nausea.

Drugs can also create nutritional deficiencies. Diuretics—commonly prescribed to control high blood pressure—can lead to a loss of potassium and other essential minerals. These drugs rid the body of excess fluids, mostly water, which contains salt (sodium) and potassium. However, some newer diuretics contain potassium blockers, which prevent the excess loss of this mineral. To make up for potassium loss, you can eat foods that are rich in the mineral: citrus fruits, apricots, bananas, cantaloupes, dates, meat, and cheese. A potassium supplement may also be prescribed by your doctor.

Steroid drugs (for example, glucocortico steroids, prednisone, and cortisone), used to treat a number of conditions, including rheumatoid arthritis, allergies, inflammations, and asthma, may interefere with the body's ability to metabolize calcium. This can be very detrimental to the health of the bones, which, given our concern about osteoporosis, is a serious matter. In certain instances, steroids may have to be taken on a long-term basis, so it's sensible to boost calcium intake with increased consumption of milk and dairy products at the same time.

# CAFFEINE

Caffeine has a powerful stimulating effect on the central nervous system. On the one hand, it can result in heightened alertness and quicker reactions; on the other, it can cause increased heart rate and elevated blood pressure. In very large doses caffeine's side effects become even worse, and include dizziness, insomnia, acid stomach, shakiness, nausea, and irritability.

My best advice is to avoid caffeine as much as you can. A classic Stanford University study conducted in the late sixties showed that caffeine can be habit-forming. And there is such a thing as a caffeine-rebound effect that results in severe headaches. This is observed mostly among people who drink large amounts of coffee during their working week and very little on the weekends. The symptoms are weekend headaches and a lethargic feeling that stems from the body's craving for the caffeine it isn't getting.

A few years ago the FDA advised pregnant women not to drink caffeine, because caffeine given to pregnant rats caused birth defects. However, new research has shown that caffeine has no effect on the outcome of pregnancy.

So where does that leave us? Taking all things into consideration, I would still say steer clear of caffeine as much as possible, but don't be fearful of the odd one or two cups of coffee or tea a day: if you're drinking over five or six cups a day, however, that's definitely too much. Remember also that caffeine crops up in other drinks, notably colas, and over-the-counter medications. Sodas don't contain as much caffeine as coffee (about 65 milligrams per twelve-ounce can compared with 150 milligrams in a cup of brewed coffee). But, if you're thinking only of colas, think again! According to the *Journal of the American Dietetic Association,* there are also significant amounts of caffeine in such noncola sodas as Dr. Pepper, Mountain Dew, Mello Yello, and Mr. Pibb. If you're not sure about over-the-counter medications, you can simply check the container or the packaging insert for caffeine content.

## ALCOHOL AND DRUG ABUSE

Throughout American history, even moderate alcohol consumption by women was cause for disapproval. Consequently, alcohol abuse and alcoholism have been traditionally perceived as men-only problems. As drinking among women has become more socially acceptable, women's problems have inevitably increased. Although the percentage of women who drink is consistently lower than that of men, the gap has narrowed since World War II. The same can be said about drug abuse—except for one distinct category of drugs.

### Alcohol

There's a very important point to remember about the difference between male and female drinking: in general, women can't handle it as well. There's a sound biophysical reason for this: the difference between the sexes in body water weight. Shortly after alcohol is consumed, it becomes uniformly diffused in the water contained in the cells of our tissues. Thus, tissue alcohol concentrations are directly proportional to tissue water content. Because of their higher percentage of fatty tissue, women have less body-water content than men of comparable size; therefore, women usually have a greater tissue alcohol concentration and develop higher blood-alcohol levels than men ingesting the same amount of alcohol. And there's another consideration: there is now evidence that women develop higher blood-alcohol levels for given amounts of alcohol when it is drunk at the time of ovulation or just before menstruation!

Here's the worst news: alcohol abuse among women exacts a higher toll than among men. Alcoholic females are more frequently disabled and for longer periods, and the percentage of women alcoholics who die from suicide, alcohol-related accidents, circulatory disorders, and cirrhosis of the liver is higher than for men. Several international studies have shown consistently that women alcoholics have alcohol-related death rates from 50 to 100 percent higher than those of male alcoholics.

I'd like to drive the point home about the seriousness of alcohol abuse by women with some facts and figures from around the world:

- A study of 103 American women alcoholics over a seven-year period showed that a third died within that time frame—a rate almost five times higher than expected. The average life span of these women was decreased by fifteen years.
- In England, a study discovered that advanced liver disease affected 86 percent of female alcoholics, compared with 65 percent of male alcoholics.
- German and Japanese researchers found that female alcohol abusers displayed far more alcohol-related liver damage at lower levels of consumption and shorter histories of excessive drinking than did comparable males.
- A Canadian study of inpatients admitted to alcohol rehabilitation programs showed that the amount of alcohol-related disease damage was significantly higher among women than among men.

Why are women so seriously affected by alcohol? There is no scientifically proven explanation as yet, but two theories hold strong: first, the greater liver damage is due to the effects of the greater amount of estrogen women have, compared to men, which, in combination with alcohol, seriously elevates the risk of damage to that organ; second, there is the suggestion of a gender-related immune response that makes the liver more vulnerable to injury.

Women alcoholics also have higher clinical rates of gynecological and obstetric problems than other women. These include amenorrhea (loss of periods), infertility, frequent gynecological surgery, early menopause, spontaneous abortions, and complications of labor and delivery. Researchers commonly report sexual dysfunction in women who abuse alcohol.

Overindulgence of alcohol should be a definite no during pregnancy. Fetal alcohol syndrome (when the alcohol and its effects are also absorbed by the growing fetus) produces:

- Growth retardation before or after birth
- Abnormal features of the face and head, such as unusually small head circumference and flattening of the facial features or both
- Central nervous system abnormalities, such as mental retardation or abnormal behavior

Alcoholism and abuse of alcohol also has a serious effect on women from the social and family standpoints. Alcoholics and their spouses are seven times more likely to be separated and divorced than couples in the general population, and alcoholic women are more likely to be divorced by their spouse than the reverse. Predictably, women alcoholics who divorce find it harder to make postmarital adjustments than their male counterparts, owing to their likely greater economic dependency, greater responsibility for child rearing, and typically lower earning potential.

The harsh reality of female alcohol abuse is frightening. Obviously we are not talking about the occasional drinks on the weekend, or even the every-evening cocktail before or after dinner, but the hard-core drinker who has gone past the stage of drinking in moderation. From the evidence I have outlined, it is clear that women are at higher risk than men for alcohol-related problems with families, ill health, and death at an earlier age.

## Drugs

You thought that the flower children of the sixties were the ones on drugs. The truth is that it was a minority who were smoking dope, popping pills, and snorting coke twenty years ago. In the last decade there has been an increase in drug use. With the greater availability of numerous and exotic types of illegal substances, the drug problem has spread to all walks of society.

The U.S. Department of Health and Human Services now considers the larger number of women using illicit drugs with their deleterious effects on the unborn fetus and newborn child as a serious public health concern. However, surveys around the country consistently find that females use virtually all of the illicit drugs less frequently than males. Latest figures indicate that 7 million women in America regularly smoke marijuana, or only about a third as many as male pot smokers.

But there is one form of drug abuse in which women noticeably exceed the men—prescription-drug abuse. This is the secret shame of drug abuse that is rarely considered in the statistics for serious drug addiction. Twenty percent of the female population uses some form of psychotherapeutic drugs—minor tranquilizers 14 percent; antidepressants 3 percent; sedatives just over 2 percent. While these figures, especially for antidepressants and sedatives, may not look too shocking, the statistics for women are at least twice as high as for men in every abuse-prone prescription-drug category. And a similar trend is reflected with regard to self-administered overdoses of prescription drugs. The government's Drug Abuse Warning Network (DAWN) discovered that, of hospital-emergency-room admissions, over twice as many women than men were seen for adverse consequences of antidepressants, 70 percent more for tranquilizer overdoses, and a third more for sedative problems. Even more frightening is the fact that over half these women were attempted suicides. And, from our viewpoint, we should be very concerned that three-quarters of the women who die in the United States from drug-related problems are over the age of thirty!

The emotional and physical health problems of drug abuse are quite obvious. Less obvious—until it's too late—are the effects on pregnancy and the unborn child. Pregnancy can be especially risky for the female addict and her offspring due to the frequently poor diet, inadequate prenatal care, and poor general health. Consider this list of common effects among pregnant chronic drug abusers:

- Spontaneous abortion
- Premature placental separation
- Intrauterine death
- Premature rupture of the membranes and septic thrombophlebitis
- Premature labor
- Convulsions, edema, and high blood pressure
- Toxemia of pregnancy
  . . . the list goes on!

And these are just the risks to mother and fetus—without taking into account those children who do survive. Babies born to drug-addicted mothers are far more likely to have congenital abnormalities, retarded growth, and even experience neonatal drug-withdrawal symptoms.

From what you have just read, the picture is very clear for abusers of both alcohol and drugs: when you fool around with these substances, you are literally taking your life into your own hands, and in the case of the unborn, other lives as well.

Whatever you do, if you feel you have a drug or alcohol problem, please seek help immediately. Your family physician can be your first line of defense, or just pick up the *Yellow Pages* and find the name of the nearest local support group.

# 9

# New Horizons

Making sure that you are in optimal physical health is only half the goal. Emotional well-being should be the other half.

I'd like to relate a short story that I feel conveys a very important message for all of us:

A woman approaching forty, a patient of mine for twenty years, whom I have helped through marital problems, pregnancy, divorce, and remarriage with ensuing difficulties regarding a stepdaughter, came into my office recently. She complained of insomnia, nightmares, and alternating moods of depression. She told me she felt as if she were about to explode and lose control. She was very happy in her second marriage, having survived all these traumatic changes in her life, and couldn't understand why she had these feelings.

As she kept talking, she began to make references to her mother and the fact that she (my patient) had married at the age of fifteen. I asked her if she had ever stopped to consider why she had married at such an early age and she said yes, she had thought about it and could see that she had made some bad choices in her youth. It soon became clear to me that she might need some psychological or psychiatric help in resolving emotional problems that obviously dated back to her childhood and family of origin. She agreed with me, but told me that her present husband did not believe in *that sort* of thing. I reminded her of the fact that, despite great difficulties, she had made a success of single parenthood, a second marriage, and stepparenthood, and didn't she deserve some professional help now to understand some of the feelings she had been bottling up for so long?

I suggested she say to her husband, firmly, "I need this one for me." Her husband cannot be her therapist, and I only hope that she realizes how greatly she would benefit from some mental-health intervention. Coming to grips with unresolved problems in our early life certainly helps us understand our emotions and our reactions to changing life situations as we grow older.

Psychotherapy is enormously useful in helping women cope with difficult work or social situations; alcoholic boyfriends, husbands, or relatives; disturbed children; and older parents who are unreasonably difficult or manipulative. Women who are products of homes where there has been inadequate parenting, psychological abuse (constant belittling, for example), or physical abuse have very negative feelings about themselves. They do not see themselves as worthy of love or deserving of nurturing or attention and have difficulties with many of their relationships.

Much more is understood now about psychology and behavior, and there are excellent sources of help available. Many support groups are extremely valuable (AA, Alanon, Narcotics and Cocaine Anonymous, Toughlove, Overeaters Anonymous, and Rape Crisis Centers are just some examples) and are no farther away than your telephone. Nearly all hospitals have mental health clinics where immediate help for emotional or psychological problems is readily available. Women's centers have well-trained counselors who advise on personal problems and do not charge high fees.

239

While it may be chic in big cities and other urban areas to talk about your therapist or analyst, there is still considerable resistance in the minds of many people to mental-health intervention. Do not let what other people think stop you from making that call if you feel you are in a crisis or that your life could be made easier by talking over your problems with a competent therapist. And if the first therapist you talk to is not right for you—and you must feel trust and confidence in someone in order to reveal your innermost feelings—then seek another.

At the moment, there is little control over the licensing of counselors, so be sure to find someone who is well qualified. Most states certify psychologists, family therapists, and social workers, so your telephone book can be helpful. Better is a personal recommendation from some trusted source, such as your clergyman, rabbi, doctor, attorney, or other reliable professional. Before you make your appointment, try to check the therapist's credentials. It is crucial that you feel you will be dealing with someone with good training and expertise. Then it is a matter of personality—your feeling comfortable with the therapist and his or her style.

Remember that if you are forty you have major changes ahead of you, some you may anticipate with joy (the marriage and parenthood of your own children, say), some with concern (the illness or death of loved ones). Life's crises do exact their toll, even though, as I've said, women are very resilient when it comes to coping with change. However, they can sometimes use a little professional help, especially if too many shattering events happen at the same time.

We come from such enormously different backgrounds, and live lives that are unique in their stresses and complications, that it's often difficult to generalize about the need for therapy. Listen to yourself: pay attention to your gut feelings about people and events and do not constantly repress your emotional reactions to life. It is *healthy* and *normal* to feel angry, guilty, taken advantage of, and sad, as well as happy. If you can talk about these feelings with somone who cares, that is wonderful. If not, and these feelings are getting the better of you—interfering with your functioning at your job or your relationships with people—then do not be afraid or ashamed to look for help.

## HEALTH CARE COSTS

A few words about the cost of health care. Checkups, lab tests, and X rays are expensive. More and more companies are providing health insurance geared to disease prevention and maintenance of good health rather than to treatment of health problems. This means that screening tests and often an annual checkup are covered by your insurance. Many employers have made access to health and fitness clubs easy for their workers or even have gyms at their plants to encourage exercise programs. You may be covered by your place of employment or perhaps at your husband's. Women who do not work outside the home may find a health maintenance organization to join which will provide benefits for checkups, blood work, and other tests and hospitalization; nonworking women may find inexpensive exercise programs at the local Y or community organizations that provide aerobic dance and other exercise programs at low cost.

When considering a job change and accepting a new position, women should review the benefits offered including health care and coverage for dental care. Considering the high cost of looking after your health, you should find out exactly what your insurance covers and use it to your best advantage economically. For instance, if you have a deductible to meet it often pays to get your checkup early in the year so that later visits are covered. Tell your physician if you have insurance for prescriptions and ask if you should have generic drugs ordered for you. This can save quite a lot of money on prescriptions.

Ideal personal health care is achieved through regular examinations by a doctor either in solo or in group practice who knows you and whom you trust. It is cost-effective to treat conditions before they become serious and the long-term relationship you have with your own family physician should mean that it's always comfortable for you to turn to that person when you have a new problem or need some advice for your future health care. Sometimes a phone call to the office saves you a visit as doctors prescribe over the phone more willingly for patients they know.

There are other excellent sources of health care which are less costly but provide good medical care: womens' health centers, hospital outpatient clinics, freestanding health care centers, and Planned Parenthood services. In an effort to keep costs to a minimum, some of these centers do not conduct certain routine tests, such as chlamydia testing: you need to be aware of this and ask specifically for tests which you wish to have done. Make sure also if blood tests are ordered for you that you are fasting, if that is required; otherwise the test must be repeated, which is not cost-effective.

In general it is always less expensive to treat a problem in the early stages than after it has become a major hazard to your health. This is what health maintenance is all about. It is really true that "an ounce of prevention is worth a pound of cure."

## YOUR FUTURE

I have given you information about state-of-the-art medical care in 1987, but I am very well aware of the fact that there will be changes as the years go by in our knowledge of the functioning of the body and diagnosis and treatment of disease. The statistics in this book will certainly change over time and so will some of the present treatment protocols. You, and only you, are responsible for your health. Books are written

and doctors, nurses, therapists, and dieticians give advice—
but *you* must read the books and *you* must seek out that advice!

It is also you who must make the choice between a healthful
life-style or a self-destructive one. As you approach forty, I
hope your maturity and increasing wisdom help you to make
the right choices.

At forty, *it is not too late to change.* Those of you who are
healthy now know how to stay that way. Those of you who
are sedentary, overweight, abusing alcohol or other substances, or smoking should realize that these behaviors are
dangerous but that there is time to reverse the damage inflicted
by them.

If you stop heavy alcohol abuse when you are forty, you
will probably not develop cirrhosis of the liver or other alcohol-
related disorders. If you stop smoking, your lungs will be able
to clear a good deal of tar out of the sediment, decreasing
your risk of lung cancer and emphysema. If you bring your
weight down to an acceptable level, your chance of having a
heart attack will diminish greatly. I realize this is all very easy
to say. Changing behavioral patterns is extremely difficult for
most women (men, too).

A few practical suggestions may help. If you change jobs,
move your office, or move into a new apartment, condo, or
house, make it difficult for yourself to continue the bad habit.
Say to yourself, Okay, I will smoke in only one room—absolutely not in the bedroom, kitchen, or family room. (Or, I will
not smoke in my new office.) Don't put out ashtrays. Choose
lunchtime restaurants that are known for their salad bars rather
than their prime rib and baked potatoes. When you relocate,
look for sites where it would be easy to join a health club or
walk on a regular basis. Think about getting an exercise bicycle
or a treadmill, which would be convenient and pleasant to use
while you watch the news or listen to music with headphones.

If these attempts at modifying your behavior fail, then you
may want to get some help. Find a support group to enable
you to stop smoking, overeating, or abusing alcohol or drugs

and your life will improve. (See page 239.) Or you can consider going to a therapist to help you change your habits. Many women who really want to alter their behavior can be helped by hypnosis: it would be worth your while to consult a hypnotist for help with longstanding behavioral problems regarding substance abuse or other habits detrimental to your health. The cost would be covered by your reduced spending on junk foods or cigarettes. Think about it!

Keep current on health affairs. Be informed of new treatments and research advances. Some areas of medical care are still controversial: there are still uncertainties about calcium intake at menopause, estrogen replacement therapy, some skin treatments, and the recommended frequency for physical checkups and Pap tests. There *are* great gaps in our medical knowledge, but they are gradually being filled, and you should be abreast of new developments. Check the *Notes* section, pp. 246–247, for some valuable sources of information.

Use your forty-year-old common sense when it comes to recognizing false claims in advertising. Don't jump to new behaviors unless you are sure they are based on accurate facts and sound ideas. Do not stop or start anything drastic in the way of diet or exercise just because it sounds bad or good. If in doubt, call your doctor and ask about it. What's often touted "on the street" is often mythical at best, dangerous at worst.

Finally, listen to your body. It will tell you things if you listen carefully and it will respond to your taking better care of it. Your muscles thrive on exercise (after an initial groan or moan!); your digestive tract works silently and well if given the right diet and not overindulged; your heart and lungs will work faithfully for years and more efficiently when not invaded by cigarette smoke and burdened by overweight. The female body is a wonderful creation and deserves your meticulous care.

So. I hope that this book has answered your questions and calmed some of your fears. My promise that at forty it is not too late to change to good health habits is valid and it is my sincere hope that I may have motivated some of you to do so, thus improving your future health.

I know that there are thousands of you who have taken on the leviathan task of being a perfect partner, perfect mother, and an achieving professional in our enormously competitive world of work. The rewards are many for accomplishing a level of competency in your area of interest and it is very exciting for women to reach higher and higher in corporate, business, professional, and governmental fields. But remember: there is a price to pay—the increasing susceptibility to health problems related to stress. Understanding your body at forty will give you the knowledge to avert these conditions and you will enter the challenging years of the future with vigor, maximum good health, and boundless energy.

# Notes

**Chapter 1**
**1.** B. Schwartz, "Current Concepts in Ophthalmology: The Glaucomas." *New England Journal of Medicine* 299 (1978): 182.
**2.** I. A. Abrahamson, "Cataract Update." *American Family Physician* 24 (1981): 111.
**3.** M. H. Jahss (ed.), *Disorders of the Foot.* Philadelphia: W. B. Saunders, 1982.

**Chapter 3**
**1.** T. B. Fitzpatrick and A. J. Sober, "Sunlight and Skin Cancer." *New England Journal of Medicine* 313 (1985): 818.
**2.** V. C. Fiedler-Weiss, D. P. West, and C. M. Buys, "Topical Minoxidil Dose-Response Effect in Alopecia Areata." *Archives of Dermatology* 122 (1986): 180.
**3.** For further information write to the National Alopecia Areata Foundation, Box 5027, Mill Valley, California 94941.
**4.** The American Society of Plastic and Reconstructive Surgeons will send you a list of board-certified surgeons in your area who can perform the procedure. Call 1–800–635–0635.
**5.** For the name of your nearest board-certified plastic surgeon, call 1–800–332–FACE.

**Chapter 4**
**1.** Center for Disease Control Cancer and Steroid Hormone Study, "Long-term Contraceptive Use and the Risk of Breast Cancer." *Journal of the American Medical Association* 249 (1983): 1591. See also the CDC Cancer and

Steroid Hormone Study, "Oral Contraceptive Use and the Risk of Endometrial Cancer," op. cit., 1600; and D. W. Cramer, J. B. Hutchinson, W. R. Welch et al., "Factors Affecting the Association of Oral Contraceptives and Ovarian Cancer." *New England Journal of Medicine* 307 (1982): 1047.
**2.** Helen Singer Kaplan, M.D., Ph.D., *Disorders of Sexual Desire.* New York: Brunner/Mazel Publishers, 1979.
**3.** S. Leiblum, G. Bachmann, E. Kemmann et al., "Vaginal Atrophy in the Post-menopausal Woman." *Journal of the American Medical Association* 249 (1983): 2195.

*Chapter 5*
**1.** H. L. Judd, D. R. Meldrum, L. J. Deftos et al., "Estrogen Replacement Therapy: Indications and Complications." *Annals of Internal Medicine* 98 (1983): 195.
**2.** S. R. Cummings and D. Black, "Should Menopausal Women be Screened for Osteoporosis?" *Annals of Internal Medicine* 104 (1986): 817.

*Chapter 6*
**1.** Office of Medical Applications of Research, National Institutes of Health, "Osteoporosis: Consensus Conference." *Journal of the American Medical Association* 252 (1984): 799.
**2.** See the two-part review by J. W. Freston, "Cimetidine," in the *Annals of Internal Medicine* 97 (1982): 573, 728.
**3.** Health and Public Policy Committee, American College of Physicians, "Lithotripsy." *Annals of Internal Medicine* 103 (1985): 626.

*Chapter 7*
**1.** *Heartplan: A Complete Program for Total Fitness of Heart and Mind.* New York: McGraw-Hill Book Company, 1987.
**2.** T. Gordon, W. P. Castelli, M. C. Hjontland et al., "The Framingham Study: Epidemiological Data on HDL as a Protective Factor Against Coronary Heart Disease." *American Journal of Medicine* 62 (1977): 707.
**3.** "Lipid Research Clinics Program." *Journal of the American Medical Association* 251 (1984): 351.
**4.** H. R. Knapp, I. Reilly, P. Alessandri et al., "Fish Oil in the Prevention of Coronary Artery Disease." *New England Journal of Medicine* 314 (1986): 937.
**5.** O. H. Beahrs, S. Shapiro, and C. R. Smart, "Report of the Working Group to Review the National Cancer Institute–American Cancer Society Breast Cancer Detection Demonstration Groups." *Journal of the National Cancer Institute* 62 (1979): 640.
**6.** R. S. London, cited in E. R. Gonzales, "Vitamin E Relieves Most Cystic Breast Disease; May Alter Lipids, Hormones." *Journal of the American Medical Association* 244 (1980): 1077.
**7.** The Centers for Disease Control have a toll-free AIDS hotline in Atlanta, Georgia: call 1-800-447-2437, Mon.–Fri., 10 A.M. to 5 P.M.

# Bibliography

Bliznakov, Emile G., and Hunt, Gerald L. *The Miracle Nutrient: Coenzyme Q10*. New York: Bantam Books, 1987.

Conn, Howard F., and Rakel, Robert E. *Current Therapy*. Philadelphia: W. B. Saunders, 1987.

Copen, David, L. and Rubinstein, Mark, M.D. *Heartplan: A Complete Program for Total Fitness of Heart and Mind*. New York: McGraw-Hill, 1987.

Danforth, David, and Scott, James. *Obstetrics and Gynecology*. Philadelphia: J. B. Lippincott, 1986.

Finch, Caleb E., and Hayflick, Leonard. *Handbook of the Biology of Aging*. New York: Van Nostrand Reinhold, 1977.

Goroll, May, and Goroll, Mulley. *Primary Care Medicine*, 2nd edition. Philadelphia: J. B. Lippincott, 1987.

Habif, Thomas P. *Clinical Dermatology*. St. Louis: C. V. Mosby Co., 1985.

Harrison, T. R. *"Principles of Internal Medicine."* New York: McGraw-Hill, 1950–1977.

Kaplan, Helen Singer. *The New Sex Therapy*. New York: Brunner/Mazel, 1974.

Krause, Marie V., and Mahen, L. Kathleen. *Food, Nutrition and Diet Therapy*. 7th edition. Philadelphia: W. B. Saunders, 1984.

Lauersen, Niels, and Stukane, Eileen. *Listen to Your Body*. New York: Fireside Books, Simon and Schuster, 1982.

——and Whitney, Steven. *It's Your Body*. New York: Berkley Books, 1985.

Marchant, Douglas J., Kase, Nathan G., and Berkowitz, Richard L. *Breast Disease*, Volume I of *Contemporary Issues in Obstetrics and Gynecology*. New York: Churchill Livingstone, 1986.

248

McLean, Alan A. *Work Stress.* Reading, MA: Addison-Wesley Publishing Co., 1979.

Napier, Augustus Y., with Whitaker, Carl A. *The Family Crucible.* New York: Harper & Row, 1978.

Pollack, Robert L., Hunt, Gerry, and Rosen, Marcia. *The Pain-Free Tryptophan Diet.* New York: Warner Books, 1987.

Sarrell, Lorna J., and Sarrell, Philip M. *Sexual Turning Points.* New York: Macmillan Co., 1984.

Sheehy, Gail. *Passages.* New York: E. P. Dutton, 1974.

U.S. Department of Health and Human Services. "Report of the Public Health Service Task Force on Women's Health Issues." *Women's Health, Volume II,* 1985.

Viorst, Judith. *Necessary Losses.* New York: Simon and Schuster, 1986.

# INDEX